HCG Diet Cookbook

100+ HCG Diet Vegetarian Recipes for Weight Loss and Rapid Fat Loss

Mary Nabors

any fashion for any damages or hardships that may result from any of the information discussed herein.

Additionally, the information in the following pages is intended only for informational purposes and should thus be thought of as universal. As befitting its nature, it is presented without assurance regarding its prolonged validity or interim quality. Trademarks that are mentioned are done without written consent and can in no way be considered an endorsement from the trademark holder.

Contents

RECIPES

ZUCCHINI SOUP CREAM

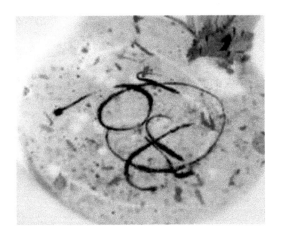

Ingredients :

- 2 zucchini, finely chopped

- 1 onion, finely chopped

- 400 ml fat-free vegetable broth

- 1/2 bunch fresh smooth parsley or fresh cress, finely chopped
- 1 pinch of freshly grated nutmeg
- 50 g cream cheese (0.2% fat)
- salt and pepper

Preparation :

1. Place the onion in a saucepan and braise until it is slightly glassy.
2. Add zucchini and roast. Add vegetable broth and
3. Let it cook for another 20 minutes. Remove from the heat and stir in the cream cheese.
4. Puree the soup with a hand blender, season with salt, pepper and nutmeg and garnish with smooth parsley or cress.

Tip :

The soup can also be made from fennel (1 fennel) or celery (celery bulb). This goes with fresh shrimp or fish, which you can fry fat-free in a pan and serve with the soup. Possibly add a dash of balsamic vinegar to the soup.

SPICY MUSHROOM SOUP

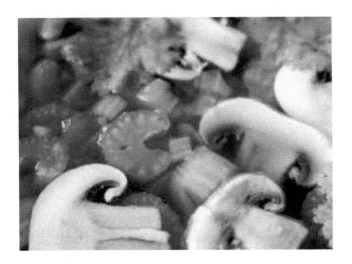

ingredients

- 1 onion, chopped
- 1 pc of fresh ginger (approx. 20 grams), peeled and finely chopped

- 3 sticks of celery, washed and finely chopped
- 2 cloves of garlic, peeled and finely chopped
- 1 fresh chili pepper, halved, seeds removed and cut into fine strips, alternatively 1 tsp Sambal Oelek
- 2 sprays of olive oil
- 2 star anise
- 3 kaffir leaves (from the Asian shop)
- 1 stalk of lemongrass, outer layer removed and cut through (lemongrass is removed after cooking)
- 200 g mushrooms, cleaned and sliced
- Juice from a lime
- 2 tbsp soy sauce
- 1/2 bunch fresh coriander, roughly chopped
- salt and pepper

preparation

1. Fry the onions, garlic, celery and ginger in a saucepan with olive oil.

2. Deglaze with a good 1 liter of water. Add lemongrass, kaffir leaves, star anise and chilli. Bring to the boil and simmer for about 30 minutes. Pour the soup through a sieve into a second saucepan. Throw away spices.

3. Bring the soup to the boil, add the mushrooms and let it cook for 1 minute. Then add soy sauce and lime juice to the soup and season with salt and pepper. Garnished with coriander, serve.

tip

A handful of sprouts goes well with it, e.g. mung beans or other vegetables of your choice.

During the stabilization phase, you can top off the soup with a little sesame oil.

Ministrone

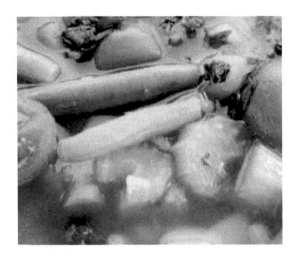

ingredients

- 200 g green beans, cleaned and ends cut
- 4 stalks of celery with green, washed and diced
- 200 g zucchini, washed and diced
- 1 clove of garlic, peeled and pressed through
- 1 red chili pepper, cut open lengthways and cut into fine strips
- 1 spray of olive oil
- 10 cherry tomatoes, halved
- salt and pepper

- 600 ml vegetable broth
- 1 bunch fresh basil, chopped

preparation

- Boil the beans in boiling salted water for about 10 minutes, quench and drain.

- Braise the garlic, chilli, celery and zucchini in a saucepan with the olive oil, pour in the broth and salt. Bring to the boil and simmer on medium heat for about 5 minutes. Add tomatoes and beans to the soup and season with salt and pepper.
- Garnish with basil and serve.

Curry cauliflower soup asian

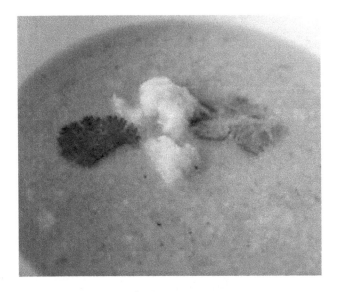

ingredients

- 1 large cauliflower, washed and cut into florets
- 1 piece of fresh ginger (approx. 20 g) peeled and finely chopped
- 1 large onion, peeled and

- finely chopped
- 2 cloves of garlic, peeled and finely chopped
- 2 –3 tbsp curry powder
- 1/2 tsp ground coriander
- 1/2 tsp ground cumin 1/2 tsp paprika powder noble sweet
- 1 knife tip cinnamon powder
- 600 ml fat-free vegetable stock
- 8 tbsp low-fat coconut milk
- juice a lime
- 1/2 vol. fr. Coriander or parsley, finely chopped
- salt and pepper

preparation

- Braise the onion, garlic and ginger in a saucepan
- until they are slightly glassy. Add the spices and roast with.
- Add 2 vegetable broth and cauliflower florets and simmer for 20 minutes.
- Add 3 coconut milk to the soup and puree.
- 4 Season with salt, pepper and lime juice and serve garnished with coriander.

Warming chicken soup with fennel

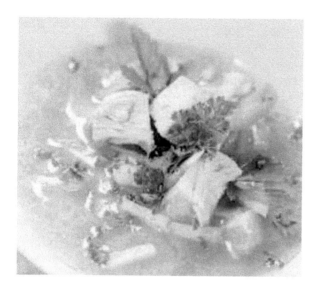

ingredients

- 180 g chicken breast
- 1 pc fresh ginger, very finely chopped 1 onion, cut into cubes 1 bunch of
- soup greens (without carrot),
- cut into cubes
- 1 fennel bulb, cut into cubes 600 ml vegetable broth
- salt and pepper

- 1/2 bunch of chives, into fine Cut rolls

preparation

- Put the chicken breast, ginger, soup greens and
  fennel with the vegetable stock in a saucepan and
  cook gently in 20 minutes.
- 2 Season with salt and pepper and serve sprinkled
  with chives.

tip

In the stabilization phase you can make the recipe for 4
people with a whole organic soup chicken. Bring soup
chicken and green soup including carrots to a brief boil in 3
liters of vegetable broth and simmer for 3 hours with the lid
closed.

SPICY VEGETABLE SOUP WITH MEATBALLS

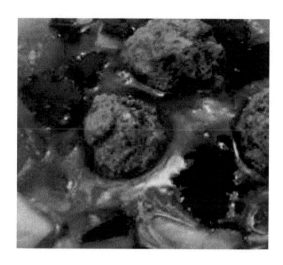

ingredients

- 1/2 tsp fennel seeds, finely chopped in a mortar
- 1 large fennel bulb, cleaned (store and chop fennel green), quartered, stalk removed and cut into thin slices
- 150 g celeriac, cleaned, and cut into small cubes
- 2 celery stalks, washed and cut into pieces
- 2 cloves of garlic, finely chopped
- 1 small piece of ginger, grated or chopped
- 9 cherry tomatoes, halved
- 1/2 red pepper, finely chopped

- 1 small zucchini, washed and sliced
- Salt pepper
- 600 ml vegetable broth
- 400 g minced beef
- 1 egg
- 2 tbsp soy sauce
- 1/2 tsp finely grated organic lemon peel
- 1/2 tbsp lemon juice
- 1 / 2-1 fresh red chili pepper, halved, seeded and finely chopped or 1 tsp Sambal Oelek
- 1 bunch of coriander, leaves plucked, 1/3 finely chopped.

preparation

- Braise the fennel, celery and garlic in a saucepan with a little water.
- Pour in the broth and cover and simmer over medium heat for 6 minutes. After 3 minutes, add zucchini and peppers.

- Add fennel green with lemon peel and juice, fennel seeds and ginger to the soup.
- Beat the egg thoroughly in a bowl with a whisk, add salt, pepper, chilli or sambal oelek, soy sauce and 1/3 of the chopped coriander and knead the minced meat well with your hands and mix thoroughly with the egg.
- Form small meatballs and add to the soup and cover and let them steep at low temperature for approx. 8-10 minutes depending on the size of the meatballs. Add the tomato halves shortly before the end of the cooking time.
- Add the lemon zest and juice to the soup and season with salt and pepper. Serve garnished with remaining coriander leaves.

tip

Fennel seeds have a sweet anise-like aroma. We can use it on this dish as it is very low in fat. Fennel seeds are rich in vitamin C, potassium, calcium and magnesium. Ideal for mild indigestion and flatulence.

FISH STEW

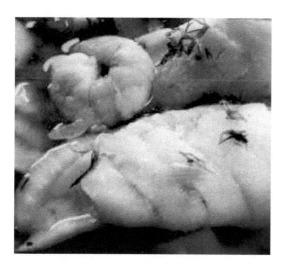

ingredients

- 1/2 tsp fennel seeds, finely chopped in a mortar
- 1 large fennel bulb, cleaned (store and chop fennel green), quartered, stalk removed and cut into thin slices
- 150 g celeriac, cleaned, and cut into small cubes
- 150 g leeks or spring onions, cleaned, washed thoroughly and cut into rings
- 2 cloves of garlic, finely chopped
- Salt pepper

- 250 ml vegetable broth
- 180 g cod fillet, cut into 3 cm pieces
- 50 g scampi without skin, washed
- 1/2 bunch of dill, chopped
- 1/2 tsp finely grated organic lemon peel
- 1/2 tbsp lemon juice
- 1 pinch of chilli flakes or fresh red chilli

preparation

- Braise the fennel, celery, garlic and leek (onion) in a saucepan with a little water. Season with salt and pepper.
- Pour in the broth and cover and simmer over medium heat for 5 minutes.
- Add 2/3 of the fennel green and dill with lemon peel and juice, fennel seeds, a little salt and chilli. Put the fish and shrimps in the saucepan and cover and let

them simmer for 6 minutes on a mild heat, turn after half the time.

- Season the stew with salt and pepper, stirring gently.
- Serve sprinkled with remaining fennel green and dill.

Asia cabbage soup

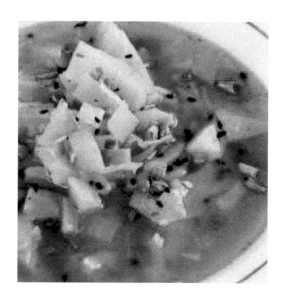

Ingredients :

- 200 g tofu, finely diced
- 400 g white cabbage, cut into strips
- 1 large onion, cut
- 1 thumb-sized piece of ginger, finely chopped
- 1 teaspoon of Sambal Oelek
- 2 tomatoes, cut into pieces

- 1 handful of sprouts, eg mung beans
- 1 clove of garlic, finely chopped
- 400 ml vegetable broth, fat-free
- salt and pepper
- fresh coriander

Preparation:

- Brown the tofu in a saucepan, add the spices and fry briefly.
- Add cabbage, tomatoes and vegetable broth. Simmer until the cabbage is tender. Put the sprouts in the soup. Season with salt and pepper and sprinkle with fresh coriander just before serving.

Tip :

This recipe can be easily prepared in large quantities because the soup is kept in the fridge for a few days.

Obatzter made from cream cheese

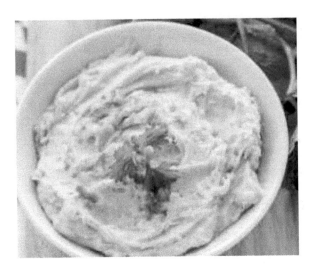

Ingredients :

- 4 slices of crispbread
- 200 g low-fat cream cheese (0.2% fat) 1/2 bunch of radishes, cut into thin slices
- 3 pickled cucumbers, finely diced
- 1/2 bunch of chives, cut into fine rolls
- 1 box of cress, cut out of the box 1 Tablespoons white wine
- vinegar 1/2 teaspoon ground cumin
- 1/2 tablespoon paprika powder, sweet

- salt and pepper

Preparation:

- Mix all ingredients with the cream cheese and season with vinegar, caraway, paprika, salt and pepper.
- Serve on a crispbread.

Tip :

You can eat the Obatzten as a dip with fresh cucumber, fennel or celery stalks or with a mixed salad.

Greek tsatsiki

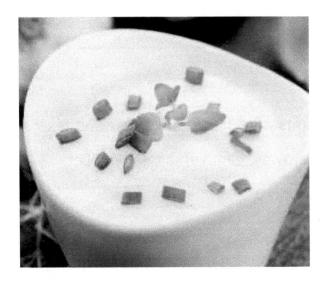

Ingredients:

- 150g fat-free cottage cheese (0.1%)
- 1 cucumber, cut into thin slices
- 3 cloves of garlic, pressed through
- 1 small Bunch of dill, finely chopped
- 1 lemon, halved and squeezed

Preparation:

- Arrange 1 cucumber in a circle on a plate.

- Mix 2 garlic, dill, lemon and cottage cheese.

- Season with salt and pepper, sprinkle with dill and serve with the cucumber.

Italian dip

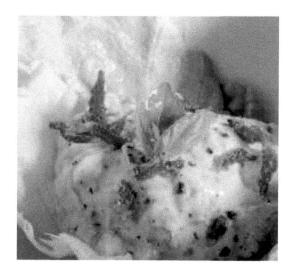

ingredients

- 50 g low-fat cream cheese

- 10 g of dried tomatoes

- few leaves of fresh basil

- 1 pinch of cayenne pepper

- Salt and fresh pepper

preparation

Mix the cream cheese with a little water until smooth. Finely chop the dried tomatoes, finely chop the basil, add salt and stir. Season with fresh pepper from the grinder and garnish with basil leaves.

tip

Goes well with salad, vegetables or meat

Salad nicoise

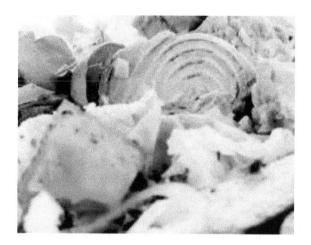

Ingredients :

- 100 g of tuna in Lake 1 egg
- Salad:
- 50 g iceberg lettuce or green lettuce, washed, spun and plucked into bite-sized pieces
- 1/2 cucumber, sliced 1 tomato, cut into cubes
- Depending on your taste, half a white onion, cut into fine rings 150 ml vegetable broth
- 2 tbsp apple cider vinegar

- 2 tbsp lemon juice 1⁄4 tsp dijon mustard cayenne pepper
- salt
- possibly sweetener

Preparation :

- For the French Dressing, mix the vegetable broth, apple cider vinegar and lemon juice in a saucepan, add the Dijon mustard and the spices and briefly heat up and let cool again.
- Boil eggs in water for 5 minutes, halve (use only one half, use the other for a later meal), cool and quarter the rest of the eggs.
- Make the salad with the French dressing. Add tomatoes and cucumber and mix well.
- Garnish with tuna, egg and, if necessary, onions.

Salad with marinated beef

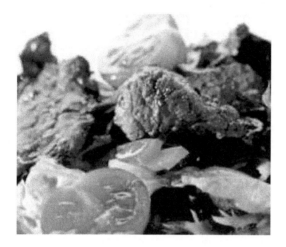

Ingredients :

- 100 g tender beef for quick frying, sliced
- 1 red onion, sliced into rings 50 g arugula and a little mixed green salad

- 4 small tomatoes, sliced

- optionally: 5 radishes, sliced, a piece of red bell pepper,
- 1 small piece of cucumber or celery
- 1 tbsp lemon juice
- 1 tbsp apple cider vinegar
- possibly 1 pinch of dried thyme
- 1 tbsp vegetable broth
- salt and pepper

Preparation :

- Mix 1 lemon juice, vegetable broth, thyme and pepper into a marinade and put the meat in it overnight.
- Put 2 arugula on a plate and arrange with tomatoes, onions and * cucumber or celery.

- Fry the meat with the marinade in a coated pan for six minutes, then salt. Arrange the meat on the salad.
- Bring the roast stock to the boil with some vegetable stock, deglaze with vinegar and drizzle over the salad.

Salad with spicy chicken and tofu dressing

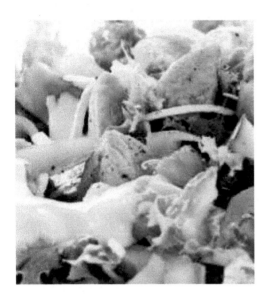

Ingredients :

- 2 small chicken fillets à 100 g
- 1 frisée or romaine lettuce, washed and plucked into
  bite-size pieces of your choice 2 small tomatoes,
  quartered, cucumber and bell pepper, finely chopped
  1/2 bunch fresh coriander, washed, shaken dry,
  leaves plucked
- 1 tsp chili powder

dressing

- 200 g tofu
- 1 lime, pressed
- 1 tsp Sambal Oelek
- 1 clove of garlic, pressed through

Preparation :

- For the salad dressing, add the garlic, lime juice, tofu and Sambal Oelek to a tall mixing bowl and mix with the hand blender.
- Wash 2 chicken fillets, dry with kitchen paper and cut lengthways and sprinkle with chili powder. Fry for 3 minutes on each side in a non-stick pan.
- Put the salad with cucumber and bell pepper (tomatoes of your choice) in a bowl and mix with the dressing.
- Cut 4 chicken fillets into strips or pieces and pour the fresh coriander over the salad.

Tip :

In the stabilization phase, you can refine the salad with 2-3 tablespoons of olive oil.

Asparagus salad

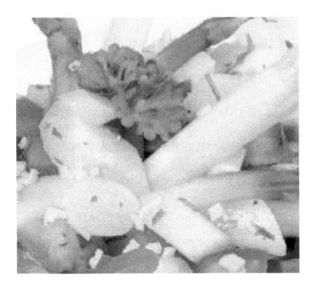

Ingredients :

- 3 sticks each of white and green asparagus, cut into pieces
- tbsp lemon juice 100 g arugula salad, cut into bite-size pieces
- 1 tomato, cut into small pieces 1 tbsp red onion, finely chopped

dressing

- 1 tablespoon of lemon juice
- 1 tablespoon of raspberry or light balsamic vinegar (without sugar)
- salt and pepper
- sweetener

Preparation:

- Put the peeled and cut asparagus in the lemon juice for 10 minutes and then cook until they are firm to the bite.
- Mix the ingredients for the dressing and season with salt and pepper and sweetener.
- Put 3 asparagus, lettuce and tomato in a bowl and mix with the dressing.

Tip :

If you would like to combine it with meat, you can eat two slices of turkey fillet.

Strawberry-Asparagus-Arugula Salad

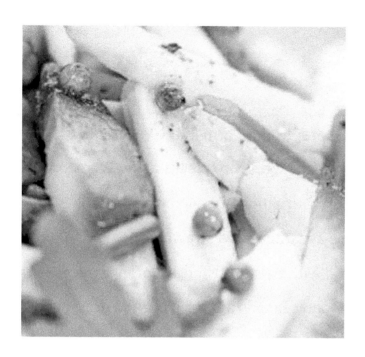

Ingredients :

- 1 bunch of arugula, approx. 250 g
- 500 g of white or green asparagus, peeled
- 1 bunch of basil, cut into fine strips
- 500 g of strawberries, cleaned and quartered 3 tablespoons of white balsamic vinegar
- 2 tablespoons. Orange juice, freshly squeezed
- 200 ml vegetable broth,
- salt and pepper

Preparation :

- Cook the asparagus until firm in the vegetable broth. Then cut the asparagus into pieces about 2 cm long.
- Wash and dry 2 arugula. Place in a flat salad bowl and top with the asparagus and strawberries.
- Mix the basil with balsamic vinegar, orange juice, salt and pepper and season to taste. Pour the dressing over the salad.

Tip :

For the stabilization phase, you can enrich the salad with 50 g grated parmesan, 5 tablespoons of olive oil and 4 tablespoons of roasted pine nuts.

Stuffed zucchini

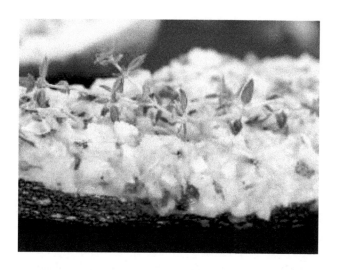

Ingredients :

2 zucchini, approx. 300g each

1 medium-sized onion, finely diced

2 cloves of garlic, pressed through

2 tbsp dried tarragon, finely chopped

100 g low-fat cream cheese

salt and pepper

Preparation :

Preheat 1 oven to 180 ° C.

Wash 2 zucchini and cut in half lengthways. Carefully erode. Place the zucchini halves in a fire-proof form.

3 Dice the pulp.

Braise 4 onions and garlic in a pan. Add the zucchini cubes and braise gently in 5 minutes.

Stir in 5 cream cheese and season with salt, pepper and tarragon.

6 Pour the mixture into the zucchini halves and at 180 ° C for about 30 minutes

Cook in the oven.

Tip :

During the stabilization phase, the zucchini can also be prepared with a little olive oil, finely chopped carrots and flaked almonds. The tarragon gives this dish a refined note.

Green asparagus with egg and puree

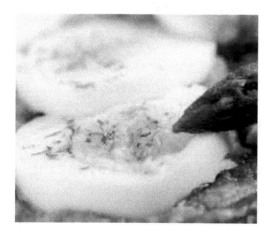

Ingredients :

600 g green asparagus, cleaned and the ends cut off

3 tbsp low-fat cream cheese (0.2% fat) salt and pepper

2 organic eggs

Preparation :

Blanch 1 asparagus in plenty of salted water for 2-3 minutes and briefly quench in cold water.

Boil the eggs until soft. Mix 5 stalks of asparagus with cream cheese, salt and pepper with the hand blender.

Arrange 3 puree on two plates, add the asparagus and the eggs. Salt, pepper and serve immediately.

Indian spinach with egg

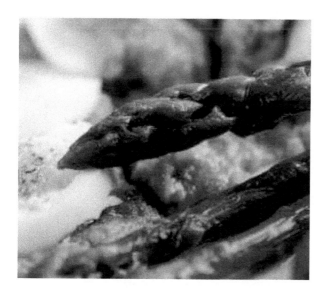

Ingredients :

150 g spinach

leaves (frozen, portioned) 1 small clove of garlic, finely chopped

1 small onion, finely chopped

1 small. Piece of fresh ginger, finely chopped 50 ml of fat-free vegetable broth

1 pinch of cumin

1 pinch of paprika powder, sweet

1/4 tsp curry powder

salt and pepper

2 egg whites

1 egg yolk

Preparation :

Braise 1 onion, garlic and ginger in a saucepan with a little broth.

2 Add the spices and the remaining vegetable stock (not too much, it should never become too liquid).

3 Add the frozen spinach and heat slowly.

4 Season with salt and pepper.

Whisk 5 egg whites and egg yolks and fry, salt and pepper in a non-fat pan.

Arrange 6 spinach on a plate and serve with the eggs.

Indian spinach with egg

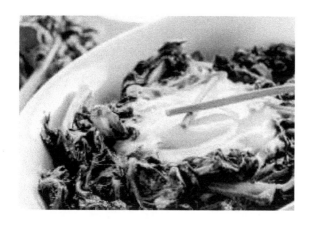

Ingredients :

150 g spinach

leaves (frozen, portioned) 1 small clove of garlic, finely chopped

1 small onion, finely chopped

1 small. Piece of fresh ginger, finely chopped 50 ml of fat-free vegetable broth

1 pinch of cumin

1 pinch of paprika powder, sweet

1/4 tsp curry powder

salt and pepper

2 egg whites

1 egg yolk

Preparation :

Braise 1 onion, garlic and ginger in a saucepan with a little broth.

Add the spices and the remaining vegetable stock (not too much, it should never become too liquid).

Add the frozen spinach and heat slowly.

Season with salt and pepper.

Whisk 5 egg whites and egg yolks and fry, salt and pepper in a non-fat pan.

Arrange 6 spinach on a plate and serve with the eggs.

Watercress and cucumber drink

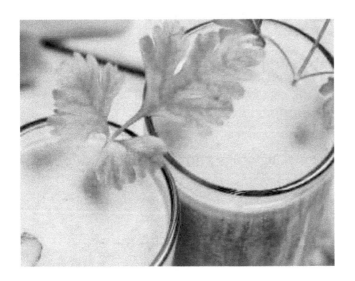

Ingredients:

1 cucumber, seeded and cut into cubes

1 box of garden cress

2 tsp paprika powder, mild

200 ml low-fat or low-fat curd cheese

salt and pepper

2-3 ice cubes

Preparation :

Cut off 1 garden cress with scissors, keep a small remnant for garnish and put in a blender together with the cucumber.

3 Put the remaining ingredients in the blender and puree with the ice cubes.

4 Fill in glasses and garnish with some cress.

Zucchini Salad

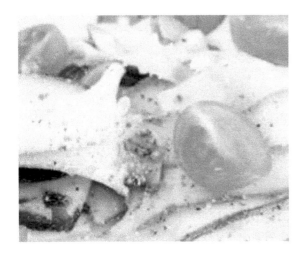

Ingredients :

1 zucchini

4 small tomatoes

1 1/2 tbsp white balsamic vinegar

2 tbsp vegetable broth

1 pinch of cayenne pepper

Herbs of your choice, cut into small pieces

salt

Preparation :

Wash 1 zucchini, clean, halve lengthways and cut into thin slices with an asparagus peeler or vegetable slicer.

Wash and quarter 2 tomatoes and put them together with the zucchini strips in a small bowl.

Mix 3 vinegar, broth, salt and cayenne pepper and pour over the salad together with the herbs.

Tip :

In the stabilization phase, you can add olive oil to the dressing and sprinkle planed parmesan over it. Goes well with meat or fish.

Asparagus salad with apple

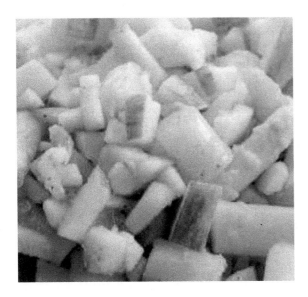

ingredients

200 g fresh white asparagus, peeled and cut into pieces (36 kcal)

1 apple, diced (52 kcal)

4 tablespoons of lemon juice (40 kcal)

1 teaspoon of curry

1 pinch of cinnamon

1 pinch of cardamom

1 pinch of nutmeg

1 pinch of erythritol

Salt and pepper (0 kcal)

preparation

Cook the asparagus pieces until bite-proof and cool.

Mix the apple cubes with lemon juice and the spices, salt and pepper and - if necessary - season with a pinch of erythritol.

Carefully mix in the asparagus pieces and leave in the fridge for 10 minutes.

Spanish fennel pan

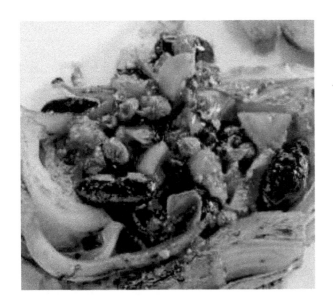

ingredients

4 medium-sized fennel bulbs, stems cut out and sliced

3 sprays of olive oil

3 cloves of garlic, sliced

1 organic lemon, zest and zest

2 tbsp red wine vinegar

1 tomato, cut into small cubes

150 ml vegetable broth

1 tbsp capers, from the glass

12 black olives, seeded and halved

1 tbsp fresh thyme, leaves plucked

3 tsp erythritol

salt and pepper

preparation

Fry the slices of fennel in a large, coated pan with olive oil. Turn after a few minutes and briefly fry the garlic slices. Fennel should be nicely browned. Salt, pepper and remove from the pan.

Put the lemon and vinegar in the same pan and bring to a boil. Then add the tomato cubes with 100 ml of vegetable broth, capers, olives, the thyme, erythritol, salt and pepper. Bring to the boil briefly, then put the fennel back in the pan.

Add the vegetable broth and let the fennel simmer for another 10 minutes with the lid closed. The fennel should be tender and the sauce should be thick.

Spread the fennel evenly on the plates. Pour the sauce and the grated lemon zest over it and serve.

Summer salad with grilled mushrooms

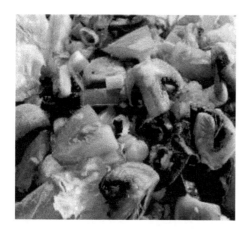

ingredients

100 g mushrooms, cleaned and quartered (

approx. 15 kcal) 100 g snake cucumber, cut into small

pieces (approx. 12 kcal)

1 clove of garlic, finely chopped

1 tomato cut into pieces (approx. 70 g, 12 kcal) a

little fresh dill (approx. 5 g, 3 kcal)

1 spring onion cut into rings (approx. 30 g, 10 kcal)

50 g mixed leaf salads, washed (6 kcal)

1 tablespoon of lemon juice (approx. 8 ml, 8 kcal)

1 spray of olive oil

salt and pepper (0 kcal)

preparation

Puree the cucumber and garlic and mix with the dill, lemon juice, salt and pepper.

Mix the tomato and spring onion with the leaf salads and dress with the cucumber sauce. Season with salt and pepper.

Heat the pan. Fry the mushrooms with olive oil for a few minutes and pour over the salad.

Fast noodle salad, Asian

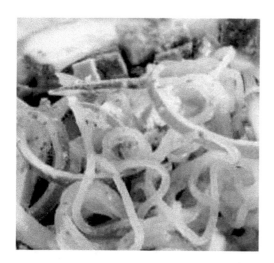

ingredients

150 g Shirataki noodles (available in the Asia shop)

100 g smoked tofu, cut into cubes

1 small mild onion, peeled and finely chopped into rings

1/2 cucumber, washed and cut into thin slices

Possibly. Depending on your taste, some chili flakes or 1 teaspoon of Sambal Oelek

4 tbsp low-fat coconut milk

some soy sauce, depending on your taste

salt and pepper

preparation

Place the shirataki noodles in a sieve and rinse thoroughly with water. Pour boiling water over the package and leave for 5 minutes.

Strain briefly under cold water and drain in a sieve.

Salt the cucumber slices and let them steep for 5 minutes. Then remove excess water and place in a bowl.

Add the tofu with the remaining ingredients to the cucumber and mix well. Season with salt, pepper and soy sauce.

tip

This salad tastes both warm and cold.

Cucumber and radish salad

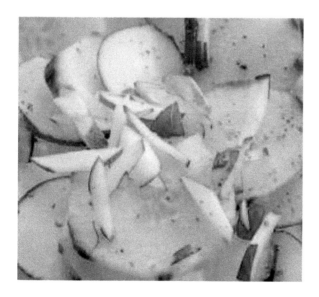

ingredients

150 g cucumber, cut into thin slices

4 medium-sized radishes, finely sliced

2 teaspoons of apple cider vinegar

1 teaspoon of lemon juice

1 teaspoon of onion, finely chopped

chili flake

sweetener

salt and pepper

preparation

Mix all ingredients and let them steep in the fridge for at least 10 minutes.

Season again with salt and pepper and sprinkle with chilli flakes, eat cold.

Yellow vegetable curry

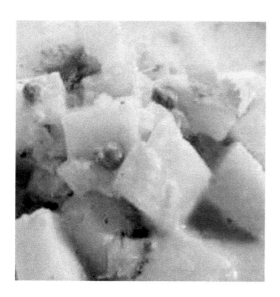

ingredients

300 g celery, cut into cubes

2 shallots, finely diced

1 chili pepper, without seeds, finely chopped

1-2 garlic cloves, finely chopped

1 small piece of fresh ginger, finely chopped

1 tbsp lime juice

100 g low-fat coconut milk

1 tbsp good curry powder (curry should be as fresh as possible. Old curry powder loses its taste)

1/2 tsp green pepper from a jar

Salt pepper

1/2 bunch fresh coriander, leaves plucked

preparation

Sauté the shallots, chilli, garlic and the celery cubes in a pan for about two minutes.

Add coconut milk and bring to the boil briefly. Then reduce the heat.

Add green pepper, curry powder and ginger and continue to simmer for 10 minutes.

Season with salt, pepper and lime juice. Garnish with coriander leaves.

OMELETTE WITH HERBS

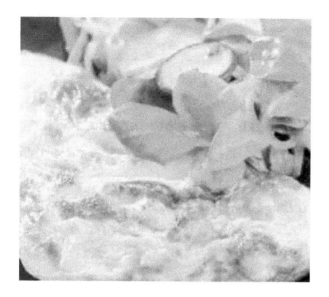

Ingredients :

2 egg whites

1 egg yolk

Herbs of your choice, e.g. 1/2 bunch of chives, cut into fine rolls

1/2 small onion or 2 stems of spring onions, finely chopped

1 tsp cottage cheese

Preparation:

Whisk 1 egg whites and egg yolks with a whisk.

Stir 2 herbs, onion and cottage cheese into the egg mixture and

Fry to an omelet in a pan.

Tip :

You can also combine this omelette with green asparagus, dried tomatoes and many other ingredients. A mixed salad goes well with this.

Summer salad with grilled turkey

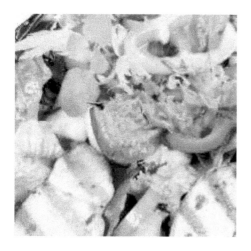

Ingredients:

100 g turkey steak

100 g cucumber, diced

a small piece of yellow or red bell pepper of your choice, cut into fine strips

1 clove of garlic, pressed through

1 tomato, cut into pieces fresh dill, finely cut

1 spring onion, cut into rings

50 g leaf salad, mixed

1 tbsp Lemon juice

salt and pepper

Preparation :

Grill both sides of the meat for a few minutes or fry them fat-free in a Teflon pan.

Puree 2 diced cucumbers with a mixing stick and mix with garlic, dill, lemon juice, salt and pepper.

Mix tomatoes, lettuce, bell pepper and spring onions.

Season with salt and pepper.

Smoked chicken breast with Romaine lettuce and tofu dressing

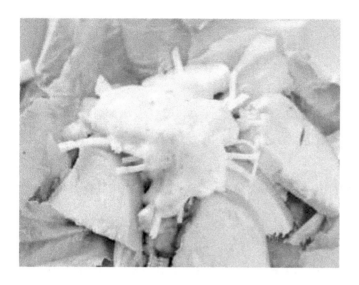

Ingredients :

Sliced 200 g smoked chicken breast

1 Romaine lettuce, washed and plucked into bite-size pieces

1 small piece of celeriac, cut into very fine strips

200 g silk tofu (available in health food stores / organic supermarkets)

1 small clove of garlic, pressed through

1 tablespoon of balsamic vinegar

salt and pepper

Preparation:

Cut silk tofu into cubes and place in a tall mixing bowl.

Add garlic, balsamic vinegar, salt and pepper and puree with the hand blender.

Arrange lettuce on a plate, spread the chicken breast on top, add the celery and drizzle with dressing.

Tip :

The recipe is also suitable for the stabilization phase and can then be refined with a little olive oil and croutons.

Green beans with roast beef

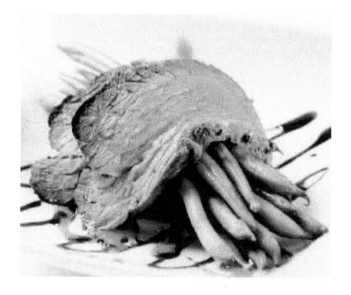

Ingredients :

1 small red onion, finely chopped

1 tomato, quartered

100–150 g green beans

200 ml vegetable broth a

little savory, finely chopped 100 g roast beef, thinly sliced

1/2 tbsp aceto balsamic

1/2 tsp apple cider vinegar

salt and pepper

Preparation:

Wash 1 beans, cut off the ends and cook until firm in the vegetable broth.

Strain 2 beans and retain 4 tablespoons of vegetable broth for dressing.

Mix apple cider vinegar, balsamic vinegar, vegetable broth and savory for the dressing and season with salt and pepper.

Mix 4 beans and tomatoes with the dressing.

Arrange on a plate and top with roast beef slices and the onions. Pepper and salt.

Minced meat with herb curd

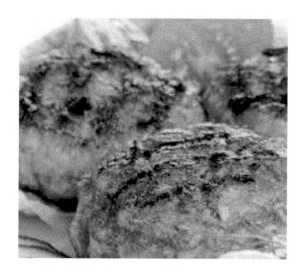

Ingredients :

200 g low-fat ground beef

1 onion, finely chopped

1 clove of garlic, finely chopped 1 pinch of cayenne

salt and pepper

Herb quark

1 medium-sized onion, finely chopped 1 piece of cucumber, finely diced herbs as desired (e.g. chives, dill, tarragon), washed, shaken dry and finely chopped 50 g low-fat curd cheese

Salt and pepper

salad of your choice, washed and spun dry

Preparation :

For the minced steak, mix the minced beef with onion and garlic and season with salt, pepper and cayenne pepper. Form two hamburgers and sear for 3 minutes on each side in a coated pan.

Mix 2 cucumber, herbs and onion with the quark and season with salt and pepper.

Put 3 lettuce on two plates and serve with meat and herb curd.

ARABIAN CHICKEN

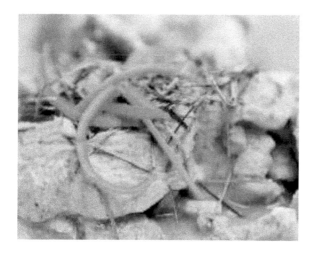

Ingredients:

400 g skinless chicken breast, sliced

2 onions, diced

4 tomatoes, finely diced

1 large clove of garlic, finely chopped

Peel of a lime 1 pinch of

ground cloves

1 pinch of freshly grated nutmeg 1 tsp of curry powder

1/2 tsp ground coriander

1 pinch ground cardamom

salt and pepper

1 bunch fresh coriander, washed, shaken dry and cut into fine strips

Preparation :

Sear chicken breast in a coated pan on all sides, season with salt and pepper. Remove from the pan and cover and set aside.

Braise 2 onions and garlic in the same pan.

Add 3 spices and finely grated lime peel to the onions.

Add 300 ml of water and the tomatoes. Simmer covered for 15 minutes.

Add 4 meat to the sauce and cook for another 5 minutes over low heat.

Serve 5 chicken with the coriander.

Tip :

You can cook this dish in large quantities and spread it

over several meals and freeze it. The spices are available in Asian shops. Add salad or vegetables of your choice, such as fresh broccoli.

Wok vegetables with beef

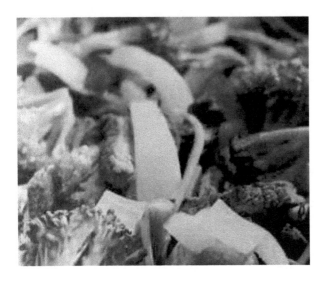

ingredients

200g beef (for quick roast)

200g broccoli

1 yellow pepper

100g mushrooms

2 small onions

1 clove of garlic

possibly a small piece of ginger

1 small chili pepper

5 tbsp soy sauce

salt and pepper

preparation

Divide broccoli into florets and blanch in hot water for a few minutes.

Cut beef into thin strips.

Cut 2 onions into small pieces and cut garlic into thin slices

Clean, wash, halve and chop the chili pepper and dice very finely.

Ginger peel and finely chop

Wash the peppers and cut them into strips

Braise the onion, garlic, ginger and chilli in a wok or coated pan, add the beef and fry hot. Deglaze with soy sauce.

Mix in the broccoli and season with salt and pepper.

Chicken curry

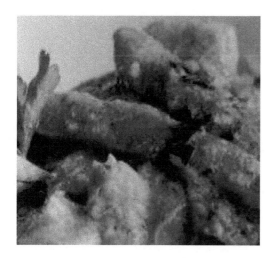

ingredients

400 g skinless chicken breast, sliced

3 large onions, finely diced

4 medium tomatoes, cut into cubes

spice paste

2 1/2 tsp apple cider vinegar

1 large clove of garlic, pressed through 1 tsp fresh ginger, finely chopped

1 tsp tomato paste

1 tsp garam masala

1/2 tsp paprika powder

1/2 pinch cinnamon

1/2 tsp cumin

1/2 tsp coriander

1/4 tsp cayenne pepper

a little smooth parsley, finely chopped,

as a garnish

100 ml vegetable broth

preparation

Mix the ingredients for the spice paste until a creamy
consistency is achieved.

Roast the paste in a coated pan for 3 minutes. Add onions, meat and tomatoes and fry for another 5 minutes. Add the vegetable broth and bring to the boil.

Reduce the temperature and simmer gently for a further 15 minutes. Stirring occasionally. Season with salt and pepper.

tip

In the stabilization phase, you can fry the spices and the meat with a little oil and refine with a little coconut milk. Basmati rice goes well with this.

Arabian Chicken

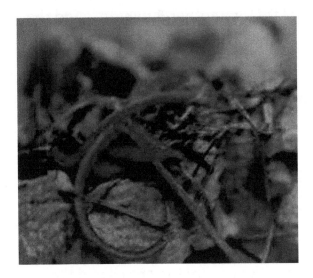

ingredients

400g. sliced skinless chicken breast

2 onions

4 tablespoons of canned tomatoes or 4 freshly diced
tomatoes

1 large clove of garlic

Peel of a lime

1 pinch of ground cloves

freshly grated nutmeg

1 tsp curry powder

1/2 tsp ground coriander

1 pinch of ground cardamom

salt and pepper

1 bunch of fresh coriander

preparation

Fry the chicken breast in a coated pan from all sides, season with salt and pepper. Remove from the pan and cover and set aside.

Peel onions, garlic, dice and braise in the same pan.

Add the spices and finely grated lime peel to the onions. Add 300 ml of water and the tomatoes. Simmer covered for 15 minutes.

Put the meat in the sauce and cook for a further 5 minutes over low heat.

Wash the coriander, shake it dry, cut it into fine strips and serve with the chicken.

It goes with salad or vegetables of your choice, such as fresh broccoli

Red cabbage with mustard chicken

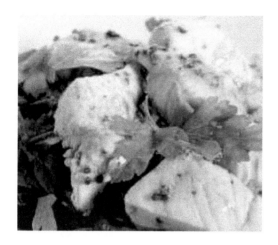

ingredients

200 g chicken breast, sliced

1 small red cabbage, cut into pieces

2 tablespoons apple cider vinegar

1/2 cup vegetable broth

2 cloves of garlic, pressed through

1 small onion, finely chopped

2–3 teaspoons mustard (without sugar)

1 pinch of sweetener

paprika powder

salt and pepper

preparation

Bring 1 vegetable broth, onion and garlic to a boil. Add the vinegar and red cabbage, salt, pepper and continue to simmer covered until almost all the liquid has evaporated. Stir occasionally.

Bring a little broth, mustard and sweetener to a boil in a second saucepan, add the sliced chicken and paprika powder.

Season with salt and pepper and cook until the chicken is done and the liquid has evaporated.

Serve the chicken on the red cabbage.

tip

The dish is also suitable for the roasting foil.

Roast beef with tomatoes and capers

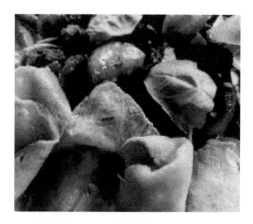

ingredients

200 g roast beef, purchased, fat removed

20 g capers (capers)

40 g of dried tomatoes (without oil), cut into fine strips

10 cherry tomatoes, halved, yellow or red

1 clove of garlic, peeled and finely chopped

250 g green beans, washed and ends cut

fresh basil

1 pinch of erythritol (calorie-free sugar substitute)

1 tablespoon of balsamic vinegar without sugar

1 dash of soy sauce

salt and pepper

preparation

Cook the beans in boiling salted water until bite-proof for about 8-10 minutes. Then quench and pour off water.

Fry the garlic and half of the tomato halves in a coated pan. Deglaze with balsamic vinegar and soy.

Put the beans on a large plate and serve with the remaining cherry tomatoes and capers. Salt and pepper.

Spread the steamed tomatoes over it, add the roast beef and garnish with fresh basil, serve.

Tip:

Capers, capers have only 23 kcal per 100 g. So are ideal for the hCG diet.

Instead of beans, if you want to go fast, you can also use salad.

Minced meat with sauerkraut and apple

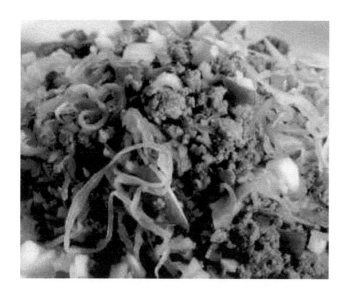

ingredients

200 g lean minced beef

1 onion, cut into fine strips 300 g sauerkraut

1 small apple, cut into small cubes

1 tbsp paprika powder, noble sweet

1 tbsp soy sauce

2 tbsp chopped parsley

Salt and pepper

1 pinch of sweetener

preparation

Mix 1 minced meat with salt, pepper and sweet paprika powder. Fry in a pan with 1 tablespoon of soy sauce for 3-4 minutes and remove.

Braise 2 onions in a pan until translucent with a little water. Add sauerkraut and continue to cook for 15–20 minutes, stirring. Season with salt, pepper and a pinch of sweetener.

Mix the herb mixture with the mince and apple. Let everything heat up again and serve sprinkled with parsley.

Florentine veal

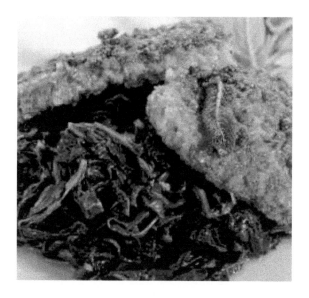

ingredients

100 g veal cutlet, boneless, substitute turkey steak

100 g frozen spinach

1 tsp fat-free vegetable broth

1 slice of crispbread

2 tsp lemon juice

1 clove of garlic, finely chopped 1/2 small onion, finely chopped fresh sage

1 pinch of paprika powder a

little grated lemon zest salt and pepper

preparation

Knock 1 chop flat. Finely grate the crispbread and mix with grated lemon peel and paprika powder.

Then dip the meat first in the lemon juice and then in the crispbread mixture and fry without fat. Add the sage and continue to roast the meat until it is light brown. Take the meat out of the pan and remove the prepared ingredients in the pan with vegetable broth.

Add 3 garlic and onion.

Finally add the spinach, simmer gently and season with salt and pepper.

tip

You can also use chard instead of spinach.

Marinated fish on vegetables

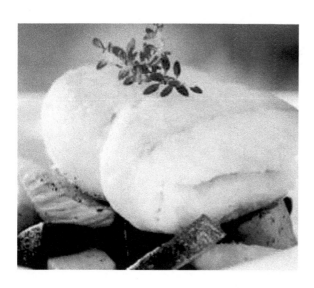

Ingredients :

Fish and vegetables

2 fish fillets of 250 g

(e.g. sole, redfish, cod) 2 tomatoes, diced

vegetables of your choice:

e.g. 1 zucchini, sliced and

1 fennel, cut into wedges

marinade

1 clove of garlic, pressed through 1 onion, finely chopped

1/2 bunch of parsley, finely chopped 1/2 bunch of coriander, finely chopped

1 teaspoon lemon juice

0.5 g saffron

1 pinch of cayenne pepper

1 teaspoon paprika powder, noble sweet 2 tablespoons vegetable broth

salt and pepper

Preparation :

1 Mix all the ingredients for the marinade.

2 Wash fish and pat dry. Three times on both sides

Cut 1 cm deep and rub in with the marinade. Marinate for 1 hour.

Preheat the oven to 200 ° C (fan oven 180 ° C).

Boil 4 fennels in boiling salted water for 8 minutes and strain. Blanch zucchini for 2 minutes.

Place 5 vegetables and tomatoes in a baking dish. Put the fish on the vegetables. Pour the marinade over and cook in the oven for 25–30 minutes, depending on the thickness of the fish fillets.

Seefood salad

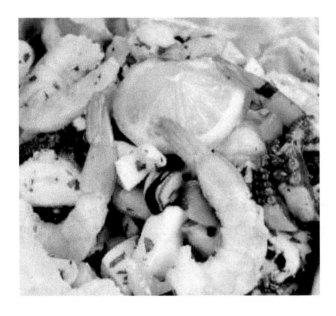

Ingredients :

3 raw peeled shrimps (approx. 50 g) 50 g squid rings, cut into thin strips

2 sticks of celery, cut into fine strips

3 leaves of lettuce

1 tomato

1 spring onion, cut into fine rings

1 tbsp lemon juice, a

little sweetener

salt and pepper

Preparation :

Blanch the tomato briefly in hot water and peel off the skin. Cut into small cubes.

Roast 2 spring onions and celery until they are bite-proof in a pan and free of fat.

Cut 3 shrimps on the back, remove the dark intestine, then wash, pat dry and cut in half. Fry the shrimp halves and the squid rings on both sides in a frying pan.

Mix the lemon juice with pepper, salt and sweetener.

Wash the salad and spin dry. Arrange on a plate. Dress the tomatoes, celery, spring onions with the sauce, season to taste and garnish with the lukewarm seafood.

FISH ON PAK CHOI

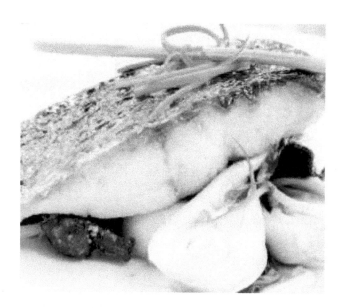

Ingredients :

120 g white fish, e.g. pikeperch or cod

2 St. Pak Choi, washed and quartered

3 brown small mushrooms, quartered

50 ml vegetable broth

1 small clove of garlic, finely chopped

salt and pepper

Preparation :

Fry 1 Pak Choi with the mushrooms in a coated pan, add a little vegetable broth if necessary.

Sear the fish in another coated pan on the skin side. Turn carefully and fry on the other side for a few more minutes. Add garlic and fry briefly.

Salt and pepper, serve with the Pak Choi.

Fish with fennel and grapefruit

FISH WITH FENNEL AND GRAPEFRUIT

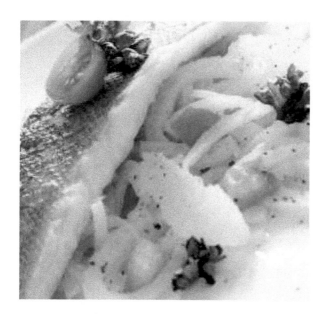

INGREDIENTS :

100 G WHITE FISH

1 TOMATO, FINELY CHOPPED

1/4 GRAPEFRUIT, QUARTERED AND CUT INTO FINE

SLICES 1/2 FENNEL, CUT INTO THIN SLICES

1 TABLESPOON VEGETABLE BROTH

1 SMALL CLOVE OF GARLIC, FINELY CHOPPED 1 SMALL ONION, FINELY CHOPPED

SALT AND PEPPER

FRESH BASIL, CUT INTO FINE STRIPS, OR PARSLEY, CHOPPED

PREPARATION :

FRY 1 FENNEL IN A COATED PAN, ADD A LITTLE VEGETABLE BROTH IF NECESSARY.

PUT 2 ONIONS AND GARLIC IN A SECOND COATED PAN AND BRAISE BRIEFLY, THEN ADD THE FISH AND FRY GENTLY ON BOTH SIDES.

AFTER A FEW MINUTES, ADD TOMATO, FRESH BASIL AND GRAPEFRUIT WEDGES. SALT AND PEPPER AND SERVE WITH THE FENNEL.

SHRIMP PAN WITH SALAD ON FRENCH DRESSING

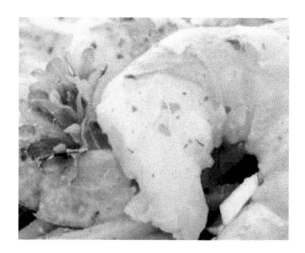

Ingredients :

Shrimp:

5–6 shrimps, approx. 120 g

2 small onions, cut into fine rings

1 small clove of garlic, cut into thin slices,

smooth parsley, plucked and chopped Salt and pepper

2 sprinkles of lemon juice

Salad:

50 g iceberg lettuce, green lettuce or other leaf lettuce

100 ml vegetable broth

2 tsp apple cider vinegar

2 tsp lemon juice

1/4 tsp horseradish

1/4 tsp dijon mustard (sugar-free) cayenne pepper, salt

possibly sweetener

Preparation :

For the French dressing, mix the vegetable broth, apple cider vinegar and lemon juice in a saucepan, add the horseradish, Dijon mustard and the spices and briefly heat up and let cool again.

Cut 2 shrimps on the back, remove the dark intestine, then wash and pat dry.

Fry 3 prawns in a non-stick pan without fat; Briefly fry the onions and garlic, then season with salt, pepper and lemon juice.

Wash and dry the lettuce, mix with the French dressing and serve with the prawns.

STUFFED CUCUMBER WITH SHRIMP

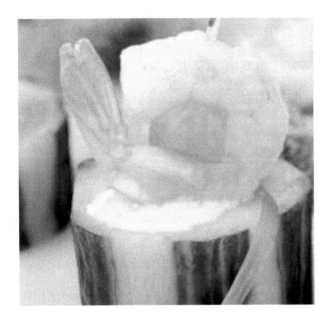

Ingredients :

200 g cooked shrimp

1 cucumber, peeled, seeded and cut into thick slices

250 g low-fat or fat-free curd

1 pc of fresh ginger, approx. 2 cm in size, very finely diced

1/2 bunch fresh coriander, finely chopped

salt and pepper

Preparation :

1 Arrange the cucumber pieces on two plates.

Put 2 ginger with the coriander in the blender. Reserve a few sheets for garnish. Add quark, salt and pepper and mix everything briefly.

Blanch 3 shrimp in salted water for a few minutes.

Arrange 4 curd cheese mass in and around the cucumber and with the shrimp

and garnish the coriander leaves.

COOKED SHRIMP WITH BARBECUE SAUCE

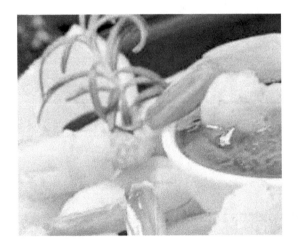

Ingredients:

240 g cooked shrimp (frozen)

Barbeque Sauce:

100 g tomato paste

50 ml apple cider vinegar

3 tbsp lemon juice

2 to 3 sprinkles of Tabasco

1 onion, finely diced

2 cloves of garlic, finely diced

1 pinch of chili powder

1/2 tsp soy sauce

1 tsp parsley, finely chopped cayenne pepper

Salt and pepper

sweetener (stevia or erythritol)

Preparation:

Thaw 1 shrimp.

Mix all the ingredients for the barbecue sauce in a small saucepan and bring to a boil. Simmer for five minutes and add a little water if necessary.

Serve 3 shrimp cold or blanch briefly in hot water.

Tip:

Make the barbecue sauce in large quantities. It is versatile and goes well with grilled meat, fish, hamburgers or zucchini spaghetti.

Pikeperch fillet on celery vegetables

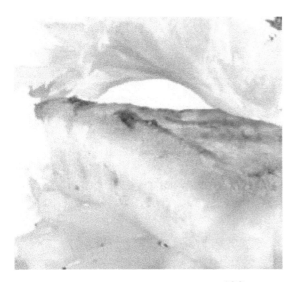

Ingredients:

200 g pikeperch fillet or other white fish

1/2 celeriac, peeled and cut into cubes

2 stalks of celery, cut into small pieces

200 ml fat-free vegetable stock

1 pinch of nutmeg

2 tbsp low-fat yogurt

salt and pepper

Preparation :

Heat 1 200 ml of water with vegetable stock in a small saucepan. Add a little salt.

Cook 2 celery and tubers in the vegetable stock until soft.

Season with yogurt, salt and pepper and with a little nutmeg

Spice up.

Sear the pikeperch fillet in a coated pan on the skin side, turn and, depending on the thickness, finish frying in 5–7 minutes.

Arrange on the celery vegetables and garnish with celery green.

Sharp shimps with wasabi

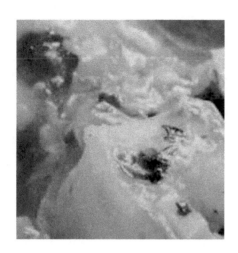

ingredients

100 grams of shrimp or shrimp

1/2 tsp lemon juice

1 tsp finely diced onion

finely chopped some fresh ginger

1/4 tsp wasabi powder or from a tube

possibly 1 pinch of garlic powder

some fresh parsley or coriander

salt and pepper

1 pinch of sweetener (stevia or erythritol)

2-3 leaves of iceberg lettuce

preparation

Mix wasabi with lemon juice and let it rest for a minute.

Fry the prawns with the onions, add ginger and garlic powder. Deglaze with the wasabi lemon juice.

Wash parsley or coriander, shake dry and chop finely, add to the shrimp.

Arrange iceberg lettuce on a plate and spread the crabs on top.

Cooked shrimp with barbecue sauce

Cooked shrimp with barbecue sauce

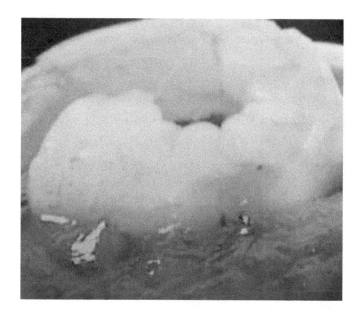

ingredients

240 g cooked shrimp (frozen)

For barbecue sauce:

100 g tomato paste

50 ml apple cider vinegar

3 tbsp lemon juice

2 to 3 dashes of Tabasco

1 onion, finely diced

2 cloves of garlic, finely diced

1 pinch of chilli powder

1/2 tsp soy sauce

1 tsp parsley, finely chopped

Cayenne Pepper

salt and pepper

Sweeteners (stevia or erythritol)

preparation

Thaw shrimp

Mix all the ingredients for the barbecue sauce in a small saucepan and bring to a boil. Simmer for five minutes and add a little water if necessary.

Serve shrimp cold or blanch briefly in hot water. Go with a green salad

tip

Make the barbecue sauce in large quantities. It is versatile and goes well with grilled meat, fish, hamburgers or zucchini spaghetti.

Beetroot carpaccio with shrimp

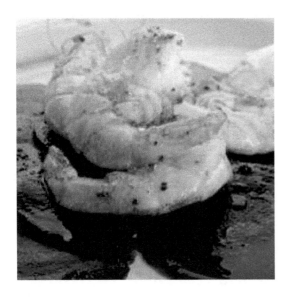

ingredients

200 g beetroot (cooked)

200 g shrimp

4 chicory leaves

1/2 orange, peeled and cut into small pieces

1 tbsp light balsamic vinegar

1 tbsp lime juice

salt and pepper

preparation

Cut cooked beetroot into thin slices and arrange on 2 plates. Salt and pepper.

Peel 2 shrimp, remove the casing, pat dry and fry on both sides in a coated pan.

Mix 3 lime juice and balsamic vinegar and drizzle on the beetroot.

Cover the 2 pieces of chicory with the pieces of orange, spread the shrimp on the plates and garnish with the chicory leaves.

tip

This refined, light and refreshing dish is also suitable as an appetizer for the stabilization phase.

Smoked trout with beetroot and apple turrets

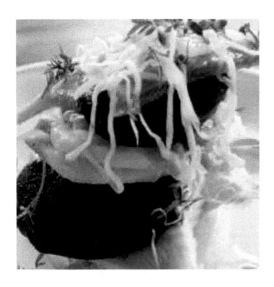

ingredients

100 g smoked trout, cut into pieces

1 tart apple, peeled, pitted and cut into fine wedges

2 teaspoons of fresh lemon juice

1 stick of celery, cut into sloping, very fine slices

2 lettuce leaves, washed and plucked into pieces

1 tuber beetroot (already cooked and vacuum packed), finely sliced or cut into very fine slices with a knife

1 tbsp apple cider vinegar

60 ml yogurt, 0.2% fat

1-2 tsp freshly grated horseradish

salt and pepper

Sprinkle cress

preparation

Drizzle the sliced apple slices with lemon juice

Drizzle the beetroot with apple cider vinegar

Mix yoghurt with freshly grated horseradish, salt and
pepper

Put three to four apple pens in the middle of the plate to
serve. Spread 1 tsp horseradish yogurt on top. Spread a few
celery slices and lettuce leaves, a piece of trout and a
beetroot slice on top. Create another shift in this order.

Serve sprinkled with cress and fresh horseradish shavings.

tip

The combination tastes delicious and fresh!

Asian omelette

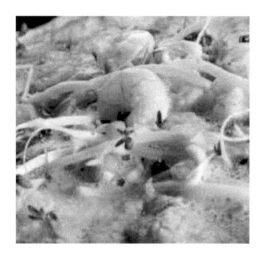

ingredients

4 egg whites, 2 egg yolks

100 g deep-frozen prawns (pre-cooked)

2 spring onions, cut into fine rings

100 g mung bean sprouts

1 knife tip of chilli flakes

2 tbsp soy sauce

some fresh cress

preparation

Thaw the shrimp

Stir egg white with egg yolk and soy sauce until smooth.

Wash shrimp, pat dry and roughly chop.

Stir the spring onions together with the mung bean sprouts into the egg mixture. Season with chili flakes.

Place the mixture in a coated pan and let it simmer for 6-8 minutes over medium heat.

Sprinkle with some fresh cress.

Cut the omelette into strips and serve with a little soy sauce.

Trout with cucumber and radish

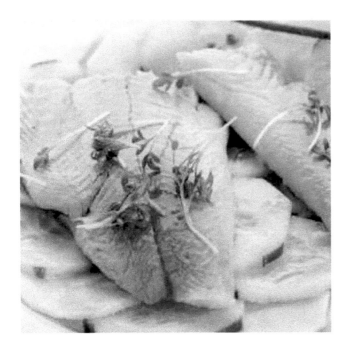

ingredients

100 g trout fillet

1 tbsp soy sauce

1 tbsp lemon juice

100 g radish

100 g cucumber

1/2 box of fresh cress

sweeteners

preparation

Use 1 fish whole or cut into 2 cm pieces.

Mix 2 lemon juice, soy sauce and sweetener.

Wash 3 cucumbers and cut into thin slices.

Do the same with the radish. Arrange in a fan shape on a plate.

4 Pull the fish briefly through the marinade and place on the plate. 5 Spread the marinade and garnish with fresh cress.

Rhubarb and apple compote

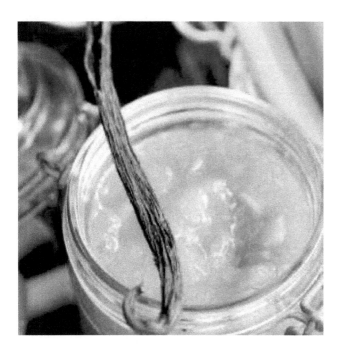

Ingredients :

4 sticks of rhubarb

2 apples

150 ml water

1 vanilla pod

sweeteners

cinnamon

Preparation:

Wash 1 rhubarb and peel off the outer skin. Cut into slices about 1 cm thick.

Peel 2 apples, cut out the core and cut into small pieces. Place in a saucepan with the rhubarb and put on with a little water.

Cut open 3 vanilla pods, scrape out the pulp and place in the pot together with the pod. Simmer for about 5 minutes until the fruit is soft. Possibly add some water.

Season with cinnamon and sweetener.

Tip:

Can be eaten as a main course with lean cottage cheese, yogurt or quark.

Strawberry meringue

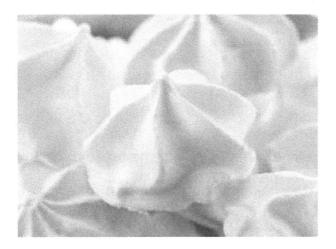

Ingredients :

16 strawberries

4 egg whites

2 tsp stevia or 5 tbsp erythritol

1 pinch of fresh vanilla or 1 pinch of ground cinnamon

Preparation:

Preheat 1 oven to 130 ° C.

Beat egg whites with erythritol or stevia until stiff. 3 Line the baking sheet with baking paper.

Use a spoon to make small shapes out of the protein mass and spread them on the baking sheet. If you want it to look perfect, you can also squeeze the mass through a piping bag.

Bake for 30–40 minutes.

Wash 6 strawberries and cut them into slices. Something sweet and

put in 4 small bowls. Put meringue on top and sprinkle with cinnamon or vanilla.

Tip :

If you want, you can mix part of the protein mass with a little pureed strawberries and make two-tone meringues.

Frozen yogurt with lemon and mint sauce

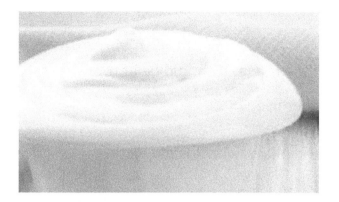

Ingredients :

2 cups of low-fat yoghurt each 200g

3 sheets of gelatin

1 1/2 - 2 untreated lemons

1/2 bunch fresh mint

1 tsp stevia or 2-3 tbsp erythritol

Preparation :

Take 1 yogurt out of the fridge. It should be at room temperature for further use.

Briefly soak the gelatin in a bowl with cold water.

Rinse the lemons and cut the peel into smaller pieces. Remove the seeds and puree in the blender.

Wash 4 mints and chop finely and add to the lemons with stevia or erythritol and continue pureeing in the blender. The lemon and mint sauce is ready.

Squeeze out the gelatin and dissolve in a little hot water. Mix with the yogurt and lemon-mint sauce. Fill in dessert or wine glasses and refrigerate for a few hours.

Garnish with mint leaves.

Tip :

Instead of the lemon-mint sauce, you can also eat the frozen yogurt with 200 g fresh berries (e.g. blueberries or strawberries).

Fruit with cream cheese

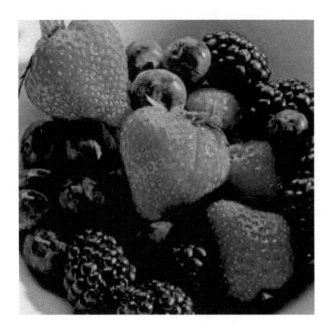

ingredients

a handful of allowed berries, such as strawberries,
raspberries. blueberries

100g low-fat cottage cheese (1% fat)

cinnamon

some turmeric

some erythritol

preparation

Put the berries in a small bowl

Put cottage cheese in the middle and sprinkle with cinnamon, turmeric and erythrotol

tip

Either pure or with low-fat yoghurt 0.2% fat

Blueberry cheese

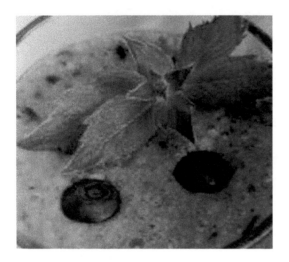

ingredients

250 g blueberries (optionally strawberries)

400 g low-fat curd, preferably 0% fat curd

4 tablespoons of erythritol or a few dashes of stevia

2 mint leaves

preparation

Wash the berries carefully and put them in a sieve. Thaw frozen berries.

Mix the berries with the other ingredients and add 3 ice cubes to a blender. Puree, fill in glasses and serve immediately. Garnish with mint leaves.

Applesauce with cottage cheese

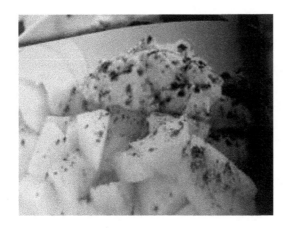

Ingredients:

1 apple, peeled, seeded and diced

some water

1 dash of lemon

possibly some sweetener

1 tablespoon of cottage cheese

cinnamon

preparation

Put 1 apple in a small saucepan with a little water and a splash of lemon and stew for 10 minutes. Maybe a little sweet.

Put 2 applesauce on a plate, add cottage cheese and serve sprinkled with cinnamon.

tip

In addition to the daily fruit breakfast made from orange, apple, papaya and berries, this is a nice alternative.

Stabilization Phase

REFINED SALAD WITH PARMESAN ROQUEFORT DRESSING

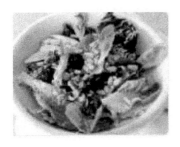

INGREDIENTS:

500-600 G MIXED SALADS, (E.G. RADICCHIO, ENDIVE, LAMB'S LETTUCE, CHICORY, WASHED AND SPIN-DRIED AND PLUCKED INTO BITE-SIZE PIECES

50 G PITTED BLACK OLIVES

8 DRAIN THE ANCHOVY FILLETS (CAN) OF OIL AND CHOP THEM FINELY

CRUSH 30 G NUTS OR PINE NUTS, OPTIONALLY WALNUT, HAZELNUT OR CASHEW NUTS.

4 SLICES OF WHOLE GRAIN BREAD, TOASTED

1 SOUR APPLE, CORE CASING CUT OUT AND APPLE CUT
INTO VERY THIN SLICES.

DRESSING:

100 G SOUR CREAM OR WHOLE MILK YOGURT

1 GOOD DASH OF CREAM

2 TSP HORSERADISH (GLASS)

20 G ITALIAN PARMESAN OR GRAN PADANO, FINELY
GRATED

30 G ROQUEFORT CHEESE

SALT PEPPER

1 PINCH OF SWEETENERS SUCH AS ERYTHRITOL OR
XYLITHOL

CHILLI FLAKES

PREPARATION:

FOR THE DRESSING, PUT ALL THE INGREDIENTS IN A BOWL, CRUSH ROQUEFORT WITH A FORK AND MIX WELL.

ROAST NUTS OR PINE NUTS IN A PAN WITHOUT FAT UNTIL LIGHT BROWN.

ADD THE SALAD AND ANCHOVIES TO THE DRESSING AND MIX WELL.

SPREAD THE SALAD ON A PLATE. DRAPE APPLES, OLIVES AND NUTS / PINE NUTS ON THE SALAD AND SERVE WITH THE TOASTED BREAD.

FENNEL FROM THE OVEN WITH GOAT CHEESE

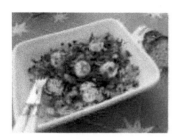

INGREDIENTS::

3 FENNEL BULBS, HALVED LENGTHWAYS, THICK STALK REMOVED AND CUT INTO 2 CM THICK SLITS, FENNEL GREEN SET ASIDE AND FINELY CHOPPED

SALT

1 TBSP LEMON JUICE

4 TABLESPOONS OF OIL

3 STALKS OF PARSLEY, WASHED, SHAKEN DRY AND FINELY CHOPPED

6 GOAT CHEESE THALERS OR FOR VEGANS TEMPEH

2 TBSP HONEY

PREPARATION:

PUT THE SALT AND 1 TABLESPOON OF LEMON JUICE IN A BOWL AND LET THE SLICED FENNEL INFUSE FOR ABOUT 10 MINUTES.

PREHEAT THE OVEN TO 220 DEGREES (RECIRCULATED AIR IS NOT RECOMMENDED).

HEAT THE HOT WATER IN A SAUCEPAN AND BLANCH THE FENNEL FOR ABOUT 8 MINUTES AND PUT IN A COLANDER.

PLACE THE FENNEL IN A FLAT OVENPROOF BAKING DISH (APPROX. 25 X 15 CM) AND MIX WITH THE OIL. BAKE IN THE HOT OVEN ON THE RACK ON THE MIDDLE SHELF FOR 30 MINUTES.

TAKE THE FENNEL OUT OF THE OVEN, SWITCH ON THE OVEN GRILL (240 DEGREES).

TOP THE FENNEL WITH 6 GOAT CHEESE THALERS (200 G) AND DRIZZLE EVERYTHING WITH 2 TABLESPOONS OF HONEY. BAKE LIGHT BROWN IN THE UPPER THIRD OF THE OVEN FOR 3-5 MINUTES UNDER THE HOT GRILL. SPRINKLE WITH HERBS AND SERVE WITH TOASTED BREAD.

BUFFALO MOZARELLA WITH TOMATO RAGOUT

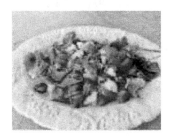

INGREDIENTS:

3 SHALLOTS, PEELED AND CUT INTO SMALL CUBES

2 CLOVES OF GARLIC, PEELED AND CUT INTO THIN SLICES

5 MEDIUM SIZED, RIPE TOMATOES, WASHED AND CUT INTO WEDGES

2 TABLESPOONS OF OLIVE OIL

SALT, SUGAR, 1 PINCH OF SUGAR, OR ERYTHRITOL OR XYLITOL

4 TBSP BROWN TEQUILA, ALTERNATIVELY WHITE WINE

200 G BUFFALO MOZARELLA, PLUCKED INTO SMALL PIECES

100 G SERRANO HAM, PLUCKED INTO SMALL PIECES

BREAD OR BAGUETTE TOASTED, EITHER IN THE TOASTER OR IN THE OVEN

PREPARATION:

PUT BREAD OR BAGUETTE IN THE PREHEATED OVEN AND TOAST BRIEFLY.

IN THE MEANTIME, HEAT THE OLIVE OIL IN A PAN, FRY THE SHALLOTS AND GARLIC UNTIL TRANSLUCENT. STEAM THE TOMATOES ONLY BRIEFLY. SEASON WITH SALT, PEPPER AND SWEETENER. DEGLAZE WITH TEQUILA. TAKE THE PAN OFF THE STOVE IMMEDIATELY, OTHERWISE THE TOMATOES WILL BECOME TOO SOFT. ALLOW TO COOL SLIGHTLY.

CAREFULLY FOLD THE MOZZARELLA UNDER THE TOMATOES AND ARRANGE ON PLATES. SCATTER THE HAM. SPRINKLE WITH FRESH PEPPER FROM THE MILL.

HUMMUS - DIFFERENT

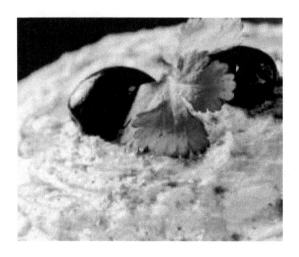

Ingredients :

400–500 g canned chickpeas or glass

100 ml vegetable broth

6 tablespoons olive oil

3 cloves of garlic, pressed through 4

tbsp lemon juice 4 tbsp tahini (sesame paste)

1 tbsp cumin (cumin) paprika powder, hot

1/2 tsp sambal oelek 1 tbsp curry

salt and pepper

Preparation:

Boil 1 chickpea in its own juice and in 100 ml vegetable broth. Drain and save a cup of the broth.

Puree 2 chickpeas and mix with the remaining ingredients.

A smooth, creamy paste should result. If it is too firm, add some more of the brew.

Place in a bowl and sprinkle with paprika powder. Pour some olive oil over it.

Tip :

Hummus can be eaten as a dip with raw carrots, zucchini and peppers. To do this, cut the vegetables into sticks.

JACKET POTATOES WITH EGG AND QUARK

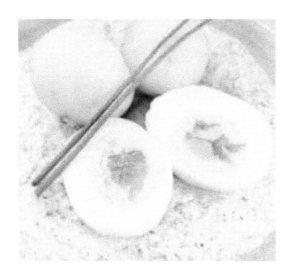

Ingredients:

2 large potatoes, approx. 150 g

200 g quark

4 tablespoons milk or 2 tablespoons cream

1/2 bunch of chives, cut into fine rolls

2 eggs

fresh cress

Salt pepper

Preparation :

Wash 1 potato and put in a saucepan with water and salt and cook for about 30 minutes.

In the meantime, stir in the quark with the milk or cream until smooth. Mix the chives with the curd. Season with salt and fresh pepper from the mill.

Boil the eggs in boiling water for 6-7 minutes.

Divide 4 herb quark on 2 plates. Drain the potatoes and use the

Put the peeled and cut eggs lengthwise on the plates. Garnish with cress.

Tip :

Variants for the curd:

Curry curd: stir in the quark with 4 tablespoons of milk and 1 tablespoon of curry and a little turmeric.

Pumpkin seed quark: Stir in the quark with 4 tablespoons of milk and 1 tablespoon of pumpkin seed oil. Mix with 1 clove of garlic and garnish with pumpkin seeds and fresh cress.

Tabbouleh - refreshing millet salad

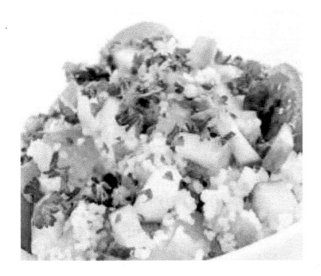

Ingredients :

150 g millet

1 teaspoon butter

1 pinch of cumin

salt

3 teaspoons lemon juice

4 teaspoons fresh flat-leaf parsley, finely chopped

2 tomatoes, cut into small cubes

1/2 teaspoon sweet paprika powder

1/2 cucumber, finely chopped

2 teaspoons olive oil

2 spring onions, finely chopped 2 tablespoons fresh mint, finely chopped

salt and pepper

Preparation :

Briefly roast 1 millet in a saucepan with butter. Add cumin, salt and water (as specified) and bring to the boil. Let swell on low heat for about 20 minutes.

Put 2 lemon juice in a bowl.

parsley, tomatoes, paprika powder, cucumber, spring onions and

Mix the mint with the olive oil and season with salt and pepper.

Add cooled millet and mix well.

Tip :

Tabbouleh is a refreshing salad and goes well with other Arabic starters such as hummus and eggplant jam.

Green beans with egg sauce

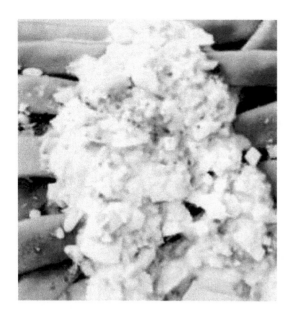

ingredients

800 g broad beans, cleaned

4 stalks of savory

30 g pine nuts

Peel finely grated and lemon squeezed

salt

1 pinch of cayenne pepper

50 g olives without stone, finely chopped

4 medium eggs

4 tablespoons of olive oil

preparation

Boil the beans with the savory in boiling water for about 8-10 minutes until bite-proof, then quench

Roast pine nuts in the pan until golden brown, let cool and chop finely. Mix with salt, cayenne pepper and lemon zest.

Boil the eggs for 6-7 minutes until they are wax-soft, quench and peel.

Crush the eggs with a fork. Mix together with the olives, lemon juice and olive oil and pour over the beans.

Sprinkled with pine nuts, serve.

Stuffed tomatoes with hummus

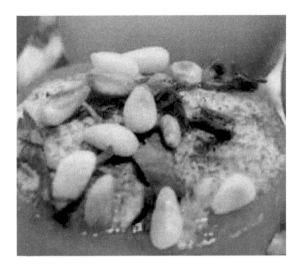

ingredients

250 g dried chickpeas, if you want to go fast, a can (425 g PE)

100 ml vegetable broth

7 tbsp olive oil

3 cloves of garlic, pressed through

optionally 1 tbsp curry powder

1/2 tsp cumin

4 tablespoons of lemon juice (organic lemon), washed, juice squeezed and a little peel grated

4 tbsp tahini (sesame paste)

salt and pepper

mild paprika powder

12 medium sized tomatoes

20 g pine nuts

1 bunch of flat-leaf parsley, finely chopped

salt and pepper

preparation

Soak the dried chickpeas overnight. Then boil in a liter of water until soft. If you take chickpeas out of a jar or can, you can cook them briefly in 100 ml vegetable broth. Drain and save a cup of the vegetable broth.

Puree the chickpeas and mix with the other ingredients. A smooth, creamy paste should result. If it is too firm, add a little more of the broth.

Wash tomatoes, pat dry and cut off the lid. Hollow out the inside with a small spoon.

Roast pine nuts dry in a pan until golden brown.

Fill the tomatoes with the hummus and sprinkle with a little paprika powder.

Garnish with pine nuts and parsley.

tip

You can easily prepare and take this dish with you. Instead of chickpeas, you can also use white, broad beans. Prepare hummus in large quantities. It is suitable as a dip with crackers or vegetable sticks made from carrots, zucchini and peppers.

EGGS WITH SOY

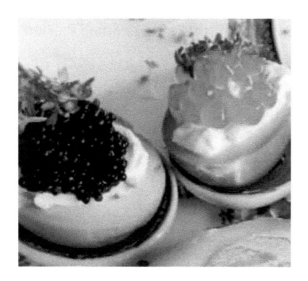

ingredients

8 eggs, hard-boiled

1 tablespoon of rice vinegar

2 tablespoons of soy sauce

A pinch of sugar or sweetener 1 teaspoon of Sambal Oelek

dressing

Cream Cheese

Olives

Fresh Cress Salmon Roe Boiled Shrimp in Lake Small Pickled Cucumbers

preparation

Peel cooled hard eggs. Mix vinegar, soy sauce, Sambal Oelek and sweetener well.

Place the eggs together with the marinade in a large plastic bag and put in for at least 2 hours. Move the bag from time to time so that the eggs are well wetted from all sides.

Take 3 eggs from the marinade, cut in half lengthways and arrange on a plate. Put some marinade on the egg halves.

Spread 4 cream cheese on top and top up with shrimp, salmon roe and cress.

tip

Eggs in soy sauce taste delicious and can be eaten as a starter or with a salad

Puree beans with melted tomatoes

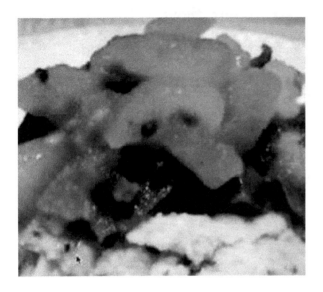

ingredients

200 g of dried white large beans, alternatively

canned white giant beans (approx. 240 g)

1 small onion, peppered with 2 cloves

1 bay leaf

3/4 l vegetable broth

1 clove of garlic, pressed through

1 lemon, some zest finely grated

4 tablespoons of olive oil

1/2 bunch of flat-leaf parsley, finely chopped

Salt pepper

Melted tomatoes:

2 tomatoes

20 g cold butter

Salt pepper

preparation

Soak the dried beans in a large bowl of cold water for 24 hours. Alternatively canned beans, which you simply heat and then add with the ingredients such as garlic, olive oil, parsley. Preparation steps 1 and 2 are then omitted.

The next day, drain the water and put the beans with the vegetable stock, bay leaf and onion on them and let them simmer for 1 hour at a low temperature until the beans are tender. Then remove the onion, drain the beans, collecting the liquid.

Puree the beans and mix with the remaining ingredients. Possibly use some of the bean boiling water to make it creamy.

Blanch the tomatoes briefly in boiling water, peel the skin and dice the tomatoes.

Put the tomatoes in a small saucepan and heat.

Fold in the cold butter, stir and season with salt and pepper.

Serve the bean puree with the melted tomatoes.

tip

You can also refine the melted tomatoes with chopped dried tomatoes from the glass.

Cauliflower tabbouleh with lime sauce

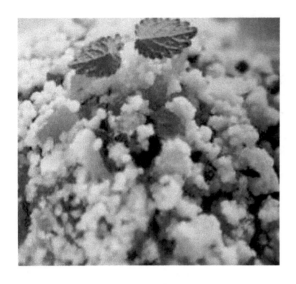

ingredients

For the cauliflower tabbouleh

1 large cauliflower, cleared and cut into florets

100 g of dried tomatoes, optionally 1 bunch of cherry tomatoes. quartered or best to use both

5 tablespoons of olive oil

1/2 orange, pressed

1 lemon, squeezed

1 bunch of flat-leaf parsley, washed and finely chopped (a little bit for the lime sauce as a garnish)

1 bunch of fresh mint, washed and finely chopped

salt and pepper

Lime sauce:

1 lime, peel and then squeezed out

1 cup of sour cream

salt and pepper

preparation:

Boil cauliflower in boiling salted water for about 5 minutes and then quench cold.

Crush with the hand blender so that it is about the size of a grain. Mix with the remaining ingredients.

For the sauce mix the sour cream with the grated peel and the juice of the lime. Mix with salt, pepper and the finely chopped parsley

tip

Cauliflower tabbouleh tastes very good on its own. If you fancy meat or fish, here are 2 suggestions:

Variation with duck breast

2 duck fillets

3 tablespoons of olive oil

Salt pepper

Put the olive oil in a pan and sear the duck fillets on the skin side. As soon as they turn brown on the sides, turn and continue to roast for a few minutes, depending on the thickness. The fillets should still be pink on the inside. Cut the duck fillets and arrange them on the cauliflower taboulé. Serve with the sauce.

Variation with fresh :

4 fillets, 150 g each, ready for cooking with skin

3 tablespoons of olive oil

Salt pepper

Put the olive oil in a pan and fry the pikeperch fillets on the skin side. As soon as they turn brown on the sides, turn. Arrange fish fillets on the cauliflower taboulé and serve with the sauce.

Puree beans with melted tomatoes

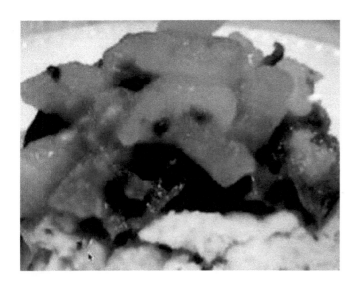

ingredients

200 g of dried white large beans, alternatively

canned white giant beans (approx. 240 g)

1 small onion, peppered with 2 cloves

1 bay leaf

3/4 l vegetable broth

1 clove of garlic, pressed through

1 lemon, some zest finely grated

4 tablespoons of olive oil

1/2 bunch of flat-leaf parsley, finely chopped

Salt pepper

Melted tomatoes:

2 tomatoes

20 g cold butter

Salt pepper

preparation

Soak the dried beans in a large bowl of cold water for 24 hours. Alternatively canned beans, which you simply heat and then add with the ingredients such as garlic, olive oil, parsley. Preparation steps 1 and 2 are then omitted.

The next day, drain the water and put the beans with the vegetable stock, bay leaf and onion on them and let them simmer for 1 hour at a low temperature until the beans are tender. Then remove the onion, drain the beans, collecting the liquid.

Puree the beans and mix with the remaining ingredients. Possibly use some of the bean boiling water to make it creamy.

Blanch the tomatoes briefly in boiling water, peel the skin and dice the tomatoes.

Put the tomatoes in a small saucepan and heat.

Fold in the cold butter, stir and season with salt and pepper.

Serve the bean puree with the melted tomatoes.

tip

You can also refine the melted tomatoes with chopped dried tomatoes from the glass.

Avocado and pear salad

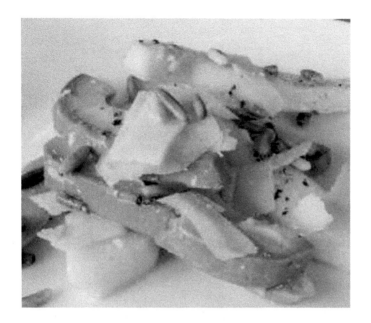

ingredients

1 -2 avocados

1 pear, (Abate Fetel)

Dressing:

1 1/2 lemons

3 tablespoons of olive oil

50 g grated parmesan

10 g pine nuts roasted

Salt pepper

preparation

Peel, halve, and cut avocados into thin slices. Arrange in a fan shape on a large plate.

Peel and quarter the pear and cut it into thin slices and place on the avocado slices.

Grate the parmesan and spread it on the pear / avocado.

Halve and squeeze the lemons. Whisk the ingredients for the dressing and spread over the salad. Approximately Leave for 10-15 minutes.

Roast pine nuts in a pan, do not let them brown and pour over the salad.

MARINATED CHICKEN ON AVOCADO AND ORANGE SALAD

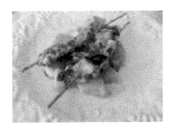

INGREDIENTS:

400 G CHICKEN BREAST FILLETS, CUT INTO 12 LONG STRIPS
AND PUT LENGTHWISE ON WOODEN SKEWERS

1 LIME, ZEST OF HALF A LIME AND JUICE OF THE WHOLE
LIME SQUEEZED OUT

3 TABLESPOONS OF OLIVE OIL

3 TBSP MUSTARD

1 TBSP HONEY

40 G FRESH GINGER, PEELED AND FINELY DICED

RED CHILI PEPPER, HALVED, SEEDED AND CUT INTO FINE RINGS

3 CLOVES OF GARLIC, PEELED AND

3 TBSP FRESHLY CHOPPED CORIANDER

12 WOODEN SKEWERS

SALT AND PEPPER

SALAD:

2 TBSP MUSTARD

1 TBSP HONEY

1 TABLESPOON OF BALSAMIC VINEGAR

SALT AND PEPPER

1 1/2 ORANGES, PEELED, FILLETED AND JUICE COLLECTED

3 RIPE AVOCADOS, PEELED, HALVED, CORE REMOVED AND DICED

4 TABLESPOONS OF OLIVE OIL

PREPARATION:

FOR THE MARINADE, MIX THE GINGER, GARLIC WITH THE LIME JUICE, 3 TABLESPOONS OF OLIVE OIL, 1 TABLESPOON OF HONEY MUSTARD AND CORIANDER. SEASON THE MARINADE WITH SALT AND PEPPER AND POUR OVER THE CHICKEN SKEWERS. CHILL THESE FOR AT LEAST 2 HOURS.

MIX THE INGREDIENTS FOR THE SALAD DRESSING WELL AND SET ASIDE.

DRAIN THE SKEWERS AND FRY THE CHICKEN SKEWERS ON EACH SIDE FOR 4 MINUTES IN A GRILL PAN OR PLACE ON THE GRILL. ALTERNATIVELY, FRY IN THE PAN. POSSIBLY. ADD A LITTLE SALT AND PEPPER.

ARRANGE PIECES OF ORANGE AND AVOCADO CUBES ON A PLATE. MIX THE COLLECTED ORANGE JUICE WITH THE DRESSING AND DRIZZLE OVER THE SALAD. PUT THE CHICKEN SKEWERS ON TOP AND SERVE.

TIP:

INSTEAD OF ORANGES AND AVOCADOS, YOU CAN ALSO USE A MIXED SALAD, E.G. FRISÉE.

BEEF SLICED - QUICK AND SPICY

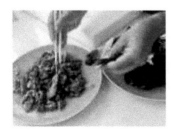

INGREDIENTS:

500 SLICED BEEF, OPTIONALLY ALSO SLICED CHICKEN FILLET

1 PIECE OF GINGER GRATED

1 CLOVE OF GARLIC

3 TBSP SOY SAUCE

1 EGG

PLENTY OF BLACK PEPPER

1 TBSP MIRIN (SWEET RICE WINE)

1 PINCH OF SUGAR

2 TBSP SPRING ONIONS, FINELY CHOPPED

1 LITTLE FRESH RED CHILI, FINELY CHOPPED

1 TBSP CORNSTARCH (MONDAMIN)

1 TABLESPOON OF FLOUR

SALT

1 WHOLE LOLLO ROSSO, WASHED, CLEANED. LEAVES LEFT COMPLETELY

LIME, HALVED

ABUNDANT SUNFLOWER OIL

3 TABLESPOONS OF SAMBAL OELEK, REFINED WITH 1 TABLESPOON OF SOY SAUCE AND SESAME OIL

PREPARATION:

MIX ALL INGREDIENTS FOR THE SLICED WELL WITH YOUR HANDS.

LET THE SUNFLOWER OIL GET VERY HOT IN A WOK OR A DEEP PAN AND ADD THE MEAT IN PORTIONS TO THE HOT OIL FOR A FEW SECONDS. DRAIN WITH A SLOTTED SPOON ON CREPE PAPER. (CHICKEN TAKES A LITTLE LONGER). BEWARE OF THE HOT OIL - RISK OF SPLASHING!

SERVE: PUT THE MEAT, LETTUCE LEAVES, SAMBAL SAUCE AND LIME HALVES ON DIFFERENT PLATES AND PLACE IN

THE MIDDLE. PUT PIECES OF MEAT, LIME JUICE AND SOME
SAUCE ON THE LETTUCE LEAF AND EAT WITH YOUR
FINGERS.

EGGS IN CRESS SAUCE WITH GREEN ASPARAGUS

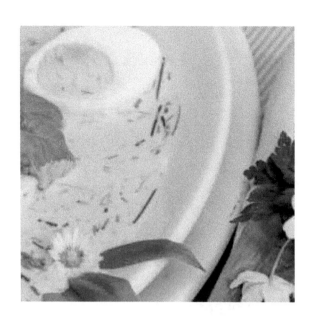

INGREDIENTS :

2 EGGS

1 CUP OF GREEK YOGURT

1 BOX OF FRESH CRESS

1 GREEN SALAD OF

NUTMEG

SALT AND PEPPER

DRESSING:

1/2

TABLESPOON OF BALSAMIC VINEGAR 1 TABLESPOON OF
OLIVE OIL 1 TEASPOON OF DIJON MUSTARD

1 DASH OF LEMON SALT AND PEPPER

PREPARATION :

PRICK THE EGGS AND BOIL IN BOILING WATER FOR ABOUT
6–7 MINUTES, QUENCH, PEEL AND CUT IN HALF.

MIX 2 YOGURTS, TWO THIRDS OF THE CRESS, SALT, PEPPER
AND NUTMEG.

ARRANGE 3 EGGS AND SAUCE ON PLATES AND TOP UP THE REMAINING CRESS

SPRINKLE.

CLEAN THE SALAD AND SPIN DRY.

MIX THE INGREDIENTS FOR THE VINAIGRETTE, POUR OVER THE SALAD AND

SERVE WITH THE EGGS.

FAST VITELLO TONNATO

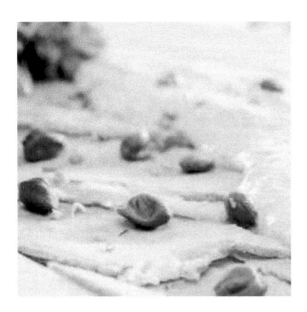

INGREDIENTS :

300 G SMOKED CHICKEN BREAST, CUT INTO THIN SLICES

SAUCE:

3 TABLESPOONS MAYONNAISE

1 DASH OF WORCESTERSHIRE SAUCE

2 TABLESPOONS LEMON JUICE

150 G SOUR CREAM

2 TABLESPOONS SWEET CREAM

50 G TUNA, SOAKED IN OIL

1 SMALL ANCHOVY FILLET, FINELY CHOPPED 20 G CAPERS
FINELY CHOPPED, LEAVE SOME FOR GARNISH

PREPARATION:

DRAIN THE TUNA AND ANCHOVIES. PUREE WITH THE
MAYONNAISE, A DASH OF WORCESTERSHIRE SAUCE AND
THE SWEET AND SOUR CREAM IN A BLENDER.

MIX WITH LEMON JUICE AND ADD THE CAPERS.

PLACE THE CHICKEN BREAST SLICES ON A PLATE AND THE SAUCE SPREAD OVER IT. COVER WITH FOIL FOR A WHILE (AT LEAST 3 HOURS) IN THE FRIDGE. TAKE OUT HALF AN HOUR BEFORE SERVING AND GARNISH WITH THE CAPERS. DEPENDING ON YOUR TASTE, THE DISH CAN BE SERVED WITH COCKTAIL TOMATOES, BOILED EGGS, OLIVES AND CAPERS.

JAPANESE BEEF TARTARE WITH EGG

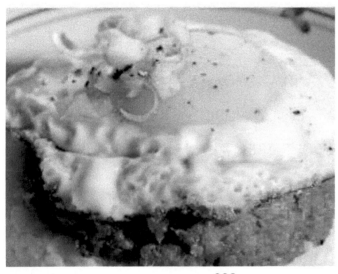

INGREDIENTS

100 G BEEF TARTARE

1 PINCH OF SWEETENER (SUGAR OR ERYTHRITOL)

1 PINCH PAPRIKA POWDER, SWEET

1 PICKLED ANCHOVY FILLET, FINELY CHOPPED

1/2 TSP CAPERS, FINELY CHOPPED

1 TEASPOON TERIYAKI SAUCE (AVAILABLE IN ASIAN SHOPS)

PEPPER

125 G SUSHI RICE

1 TABLESPOON OF OLIVE OIL

2 EGGS

1/2 BUNCH OF CHIVES, CUT INTO FINE RINGS

SALT AND PEPPER

PREPARATION

COOK THE SUSHI RICE IN SALTED WATER ACCORDING TO THE PACKAGE INSTRUCTIONS AND LET IT COOL

MIX THE BEEF TARTARE WITH SWEETENER, BELL PEPPER, ANCHOVIES, CAPERS, TERIYAKI SAUCE, SALT AND PEPPER. IF YOU WANT TO MAKE IT MORE SPICY, YOU CAN ADD 1/2 TEASPOON OF SAMBAL OELEK.

FILL THE RICE INTO A SMALL ROUND OR SQUARE SHAPE, PRESS IT DOWN AND FLIP IT ONTO A PLATE. PUT THE TARTARE ON TOP AND FLATTEN IT A LITTLE.

HEAT THE OIL IN A PAN AND FRY THE EGGS AS FRIED EGGS. PLACE ON THE TARTARE AND SPRINKLE WITH SALT, PEPPER AND CHIVES. SERVE IMMEDIATELY.

SHRIMP WITH CURRY SAUCE

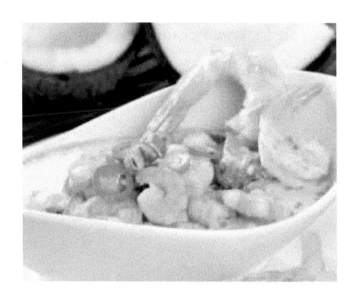

Ingredients :

300 g large shrimp

1 onion, finely chopped

1 small red chilli or chilli flakes

1 clove of garlic, pressed through

20 g ginger, finely chopped

1 small cucumber, finely diced

3 slices of fresh pineapple (optionally canned sugar-free), finely diced 1 tablespoon butter

1 tbsp Curry powder

100 ml vegetable broth

4 tbsp canned coconut milk (the rest can be frozen)

1 tbsp soy sauce a

little fresh coriander, washed, shaken dry

1 pinch of cayenne pepper

salt and pepper

Preparation:

Peel, wash and pat dry shrimp.

If you like it spicy, you can halve a chili pepper, remove the stone and cut into fine rings. Save a few for the set. Use chilli flakes as an alternative.

Put butter in a small saucepan and sauté the onion, garlic and chili peppers until translucent. Add the curry powder and ginger and bring to the boil with the vegetable stock and coconut milk. Add the shrimp, cucumber and pineapple cubes and the shrimp and steam for 5-6 minutes at low temperature.

Season with salt, pepper, cayenne pepper and soy sauce and serve with fresh coriander leaves.

EXOTIC BERRY COCONUT DESSERT

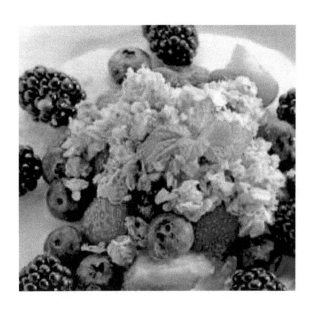

INGREDIENTS

30 G PITHY OATMEAL

1/2 TSP FINELY GRATED FRESH GINGER

500 G OF BERRIES SUCH AS STRAWBERRIES, RASPBERRIES, BLUEBERRIES, WASHED

3 TBSP ALGAVE SYRUP

2 ORGANIC LIMES

250 G FIRM COCONUT CREAM (ASIA SHOP)

PREPARATION

WASH THE LIMES HOT. GRATE THE PEEL FINELY, THEN SQUEEZE THE JUICE AND POUR HALF OVER THE BERRIES.

ROAST OATMEAL IN A SAUCEPAN WITH THE GINGER, THEN SWEETEN WITH 2 TBSP ALGAE SYRUP AND STIR UNTIL CRUMPLE FORMS. ADD 2 TEASPOONS OF COKE CREAM.

WARM UP COCONUT CREAM, STIR IN AGAVE SYRUP AND MIX WITH THE REMAINING LIME JUICE.

ARRANGE THE BERRIES ON A PLATE. PUT A LARGE TABLESPOON OF OATMEAL IN THE MIDDLE AND SPREAD THE COKE CREAM AROUND IT.

TENDERLOIN STEAK WITH CAULIFLOWER AND LETTUCE

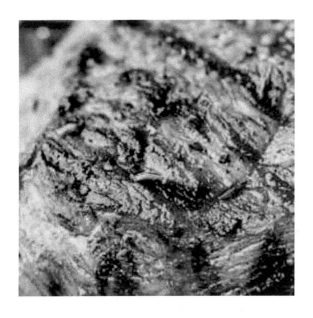

INGREDIENTS

2 STEAKS OF AROUND 100 GRAMS

1 ONION

TRAY OF MUSHROOMS

1 CAULIFLOWER

ARUGULA LETTUCE (OR ICEBERG)

CALVÉ SALAD DRESSING

A LITTLE STOCK POWDER

PEPPER AND SALT

PREPARATION

CUT THE ONION INTO RINGS AND THE MUSHROOMS INTO SLICES

MEANWHILE, BOIL THE CAULIFLOWER WITH A LITTLE BOUILLON POWDER. (COOK THE CAULIFLOWER IN 15 MINUTES UNTIL DONE.)

GET THE STEAKS AND ADD A LITTLE SALT AND PEPPER.

PLACE THEM IN A GRILL PAN AND SEAL BOTH SIDES. YOU CAN CHOOSE WHETHER YOU WANT THE STEAK MEDIUM, RARE OR WELL DONE.

ADD THE SLICED ONION AND MUSHROOMS TO THE STEAK AND FRY BRIEFLY.

IN THE MEANTIME YOU CAN PREPARE THE LETTUCE. PUT THE ARUGULA (OR ICEBERG) LETTUCE IN A BOWL. MAKE THE SALAD DRESSING (CALVÉ SALAD MIX) WITH 6 TABLESPOONS OF WATER AND SPRINKLE OVER THE LETTUCE.

YOU CAN POSSIBLY EXTINGUISH THE STEAK WITH THE CAULIFLOWER MOISTURE.

PUT IT ALL ON A PLATE. AND, VERY TASTY!

TURKEY OR CHICKEN SKEWERS

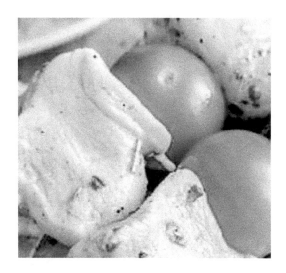

Ingredients

400 grams of chicken or turkey fillet

Sip of soy sauce

2 cloves of garlic

1 tablespoon soy sauce

half teaspoon of ginger powder

half teaspoon of sambal

Possibly a few sherry tomatoes or other permitted
vegetables

4 large skewers

400 grams of spinach

1 egg

Salt and pepper to taste

Pem spray

Preparation method

Cut the chicken or turkey fillet into cubes and put them in a bowl.

Add the soy sauce, ginger powder, sambal and a dash of soy sauce. Using a garlic press, squeeze the garlic above the dish.

Stir everything well and cover the dish with cling film. Let the chicken or turkey marinate in the fridge for an hour.

Meanwhile, boil an egg. (For the spinach)

After marinating for an hour, you can thread the pieces of fillet to the skewers. You can put pieces of vegetables between the pieces of fillet. Spray a little Pem Spray on it.

Now grill the skewers on the barbecue, grill plate or in a frying pan.

In the meantime you can wash the spinach (if necessary) and blanch briefly in boiling water. Then drain in a colander. Peel the egg and place the egg white on top. For a nice bite you can crumble 2 more breadsticks through it.

LASAGNA WITH CABBAGE

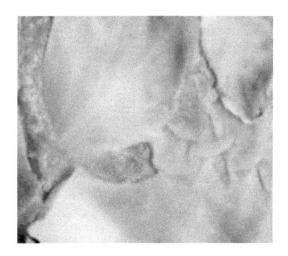

Ingredients:

1 cabbage (white, Chinese or Savoy)

300 grams of lean ham

4 large beef tomatoes

Broth

Goat cheese or mozzarella

Tomato sauce

Tip: You can make some extra tomato and cauliflower sauce
and keep it in the fridge. You can use these sauces with

more dishes. As it is also described in the accompanying book.

Preparation method

Make the tomato and cauliflower sauce as described above. Or maybe you still have it in the fridge.

Cut around 12 to 15 leaves from the cabbage (without the veins). Slice the beef tomatoes.

Preheat the oven to 180 degrees.

Heat a pan with hot water and blanch the cabbage leaves.

Rinse them with cold water after blanching. This way they retain their fresh color.

You now start building the lasagna. Start with a layer of tomato sauce and slices of tomatoes. Cover this with a few blanched cabbage leaves. Cover the leaves with the ham. On the ham you put another layer of tomato sauce with slices of tomatoes. This way you continue building until the ingredients are used up.

Finally, add the cauliflower sauce over the lasagna.

Place the lasagna in a preheated oven and let it stand for 25 minutes.

Add a slightly ground goat cheese or mozzarella.

Omelet with various vegetables

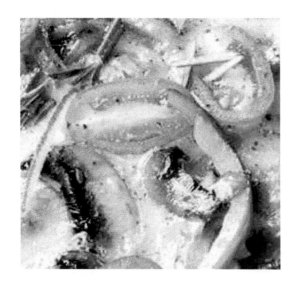

Ingredients

3 eggs

2 tablespoons skimmed milk

Mushrooms

Bean sprouts

Onion

Tomato

Chives

Possibly a little pepper and salt

Preparation method

You use 3 eggs for this omelet, of which only 1 yolk. (2 yolks do away). The fats in an egg are in the yolk.

Beat the eggs together with 2 tablespoons of skimmed milk.

Meanwhile, cut the onion, mushrooms, tomato and chives into pieces.

Add all vegetables to the omelette batter.

Let a pan get hot and fry the whole into a tasty omelet.

If desired, you can add a little more pepper and salt.

Asparagus with egg

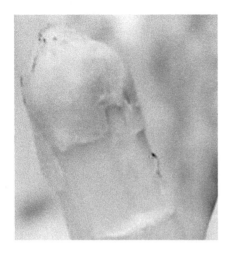

Ingredients

+/- 600 grams of white asparagus

6-7 eggs

salt

Possibly some chives

Preparation

Start by cleaning the asparagus. Cut 2 centimeters from the bottom and peel the asparagus with a peeler.

Put the asparagus in a pan with water. Add a pinch of salt.

Cook the asparagus in about 10 to 12 minutes. (Depending on the thickness of the asparagus).

In the meantime you can start boiling the eggs. Do this in about 6 to 7 minutes.

Let the eggs cool in cold water and remove the skin.

From 4-5 eggs you then remove the egg yellow and use only the protein. The egg yellow contains the fats and we want to limit this in the slimming phase.

Once the asparagus is ready, place them on a plate. Place the eggs on the asparagus and sprinkle with a little cooking liquid. If desired, you can sprinkle something chive here.

COD FILLET FROM THE OVEN

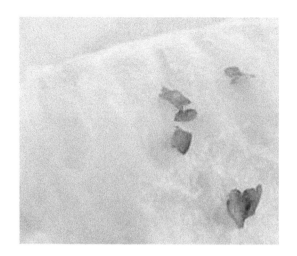

INGREDIENTS

400 GRAMS OF LEEK

1 YELLOW PEPPER

400 GRAMS OF COD FILLET (4 PIECES OF +/- 100 GRAMS)
(OR PANGASIUS)

100 GRAMS OF GRATED CHEESE (20+ OR 30+)

LIME

CORIANDER

PAM SPRAY

FOR TABLE COMPANIONS: MASHED POTATOES

PREPARATION

PREHEAT THE OVEN TO 225 DEGREES.

CUT THE LEEK AND THE YELLOW BELL PEPPER INTO THIN STRIPS

TAKE THE FISH FILLET AND SPRINKLE IT WITH LIME JUICE AND SPRINKLE SOME CORIANDER OVER IT.

SPRAY A BAKING DISH WITH A LITTLE PAM SPRAY. THEN COVER THE BOTTOM WITH HALF THE SLICED LEEK AND BELL PEPPER. PUT THE FISH FILLET ON TOP AND COVER THE FISH WITH THE REMAINING HALF OF THE LEEK AND BELL PEPPER.

SPRINKLE THE GRATED CHEESE OVER THIS WHOLE.

PLACE THE BAKING DISH IN THE MIDDLE OF THE OVEN AND LET THE FISH COOK IN ABOUT 18 MINUTES.

SPINACH ROLLS WITH EGG

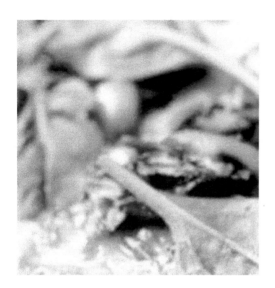

Ingredients

900 grams of spinach

5 eggs

2 tablespoons pine nuts

Pem spray

1 beef tomato

Chopped parsley

1 tablespoon of Italian herbs (chopped or dried)

100 grams of Parmesan cheese (grated)

Pepper and salt

Preparation

Boil the spinach (with a pinch of salt if necessary) in about 2 minutes. Then drain and drain well.

Beat the eggs with 3 tablespoons of water and a little salt and pepper.

Meanwhile, roast the pine nuts in a dry and hot frying pan. This only needs a moment. Then set them apart.

Preheat the oven to 200 degrees.

Spray the Pem in a frying pan and pour 2-3 tablespoons of the egg mixtures into the pan. Bake a small omelet.

Repeat this until the egg mixes are finished. You probably have about 8 omelettes.

Cut the beef tomato into small cubes.

Take a bowl and put in the drained spinach, pine nuts, tomato cubes, Italian herbs and half of the cheese.

Divide the spinach filling over the omelettes. Shape into rolls and place in a baking dish. Place the remaining spinach in a border around the filled omelettes.

Put the rest of the Parmesan cheese on the omelettes and put the dish in the oven for about 15 minutes.

Garnish with a little chopped parsley.

STUFFED MUSHROOMS

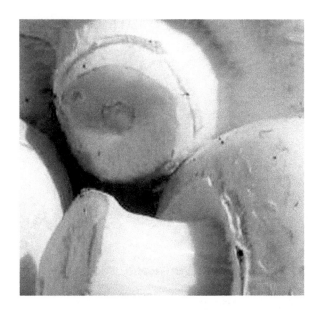

Ingredients

A bowl of large mushrooms

120 grams of chicken

1 onion

1 leek

Bean sprouts

Lettuce

Broth powder

Pem Spray

400 ml of water

Or possibly other vegetables

Preparation method

Preheat the oven to 180 degrees.

Take the large mushrooms and remove the stem. If necessary, you can hollow out the mushrooms a little further.

Then cut the chicken into small pieces and also cut all vegetables (with the exception of the mushrooms)

Spray a frying pan with pem spray and cook the chicken until tender. Add the vegetables over time.

When the whole is done, add 400 ml of water and a little stock powder. Let it stand for 15 minutes. This way the taste of the bouillon powder can draw in the ingredients.

Put the chicken and vegetables in the large mushrooms.

Take a baking dish and carefully place the stuffed mushrooms in it. Let the mushrooms cook in the oven for 10 minutes.

Place the mushrooms on a bed of lettuce and bean sprouts.

PROTEIN SHAKE

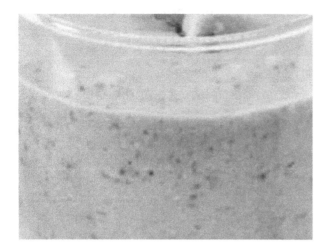

Ingredients:

20 grams of Amino fit (one scoop)

300 ml Skimmed milk or Yogurt

Fruit, for example, a handful of blackberries and red berries

Preparation

Put 300 ml of skimmed milk or low-fat yogurt in a blender.

Add a measuring spoon, about 20 grams, of Amino-fit.

Finally, add a handful of blackberries and red berries. This may also be other fruit

Blend the whole into a tasty and nutritious shake.

If you use low-fat yogurt, the shake may be just a little too thick. Add a little water to make it more drinkable.

CAULIFLOWER PIZZA

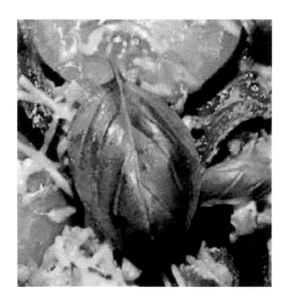

Ingredients

Ingredients bottom:

1 medium cauliflower

Pinch of sea salt

2 cloves of garlic

1/2 tsp dried basil

1/2 tsp dried oregano

half outing

ginger powder

chili powder

1 egg

1 tsp olive oil

Ingredients Topping:

Tomato sauce (possibly homemade)

Tray of Mushrooms

Red pepper

1 onion

artichoke

Cherry tomatoes

Parmesan cheese

Preparation

Preheat the oven to 200 degrees.

Wash the cauliflower and make small florets.

Finely grate the cauliflower. You can also crush the cauliflower in a food processor.

Place the grated or finely ground cauliflower in an ovenproof dish and heat it for about 7 minutes. The moisture is therefore released from the cauliflower. Let the cauliflower drain and cool a little.

Place the drained cauliflower on a clean tea towel and close the tea towel. Wring it out well so that all the moisture is out. Then unfold the tea towel and crumble it a bit loose.

Crush the garlic and onion until it is puree.

Put the cauliflower in a bowl and add the mashed garlic and onion, olive oil, basil, oregano, a little chili pepper, ginger powder and salt. Mix the whole and finally add the egg.

Make a kind of dough ball from the whole mixture. You can do this with your hand.

Cover your baking sheet with baking paper and spray it with a little Pem so that it does not stick too much.

Then divide the dough ball over the baking paper so that an even bottom is created. Keep about 0.5 cm. You can possibly press it with the convex side of a spoon.

Put the pizza crust in the oven and bake it in 10 to 15 minutes. If the pizza base is well browned, you can turn it over again (about 3 more minutes), so that the underside becomes nice and crunchy.

When the pizza base is ready, you can garnish it with the (possibly homemade) tomato sauce, bell pepper, mushrooms, onion, artichoke and cherry tomatoes.

Put the prepared pizza in the oven for about 8 minutes.

MEAL VEGETABLE SOUP

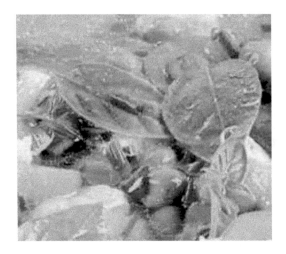

Ingredients

500 grams of lean poulet

750 grams of coarsely sliced soup vegetables

1 herb bag for meat stock

1 packet of flavor enhancer (maggi)

Preparation

Take a large pan, add 3 liters of water and bring to the boil.

As soon as the water boils, add the poulet. Then bring it back to the boil. (Remove the foam if necessary)

Hang the herb bag in the boiling water and lower the heat a little. Set it so low that it stays just a little to the boil. Let it stand for 3 hours.

Add the coarsely chopped soup vegetables after 3 hours and let it cook for 15 minutes.

If there is too much carrot in the soup vegetable, you can take it out. A bit is of course not bad.

You can add the flavor enhancer for the last 5 minutes. You can also choose to add a little sprinkling stock, salt, pepper and spices. This is after your own taste.

Serve with breadsticks.

Meatball with spinach and egg

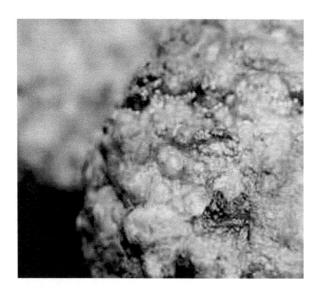

Ingredients

200 grams of lean ground beef

2 eggs

2 cloves of garlic

2 tbsp fresh basil

2 breadsticks

Fresh spinach

Preparation

Place the minced meat in a large bowl and add half an egg, crushed garlic, finely chopped basil and half a stem.

Knead the whole and add a little salt and pepper to taste. Turn the meatballs into 2 equal balls.

Heat a pan with PEM spray and bake the balls until done.

In the meantime you can cook the spinach. Once done, drain well.

Put the remaining one-and-a-half sticks in the cooked spinach.

Garnish the spinach with a boiled egg (only the protein)

Celeriac soup with a chicken / beet salad

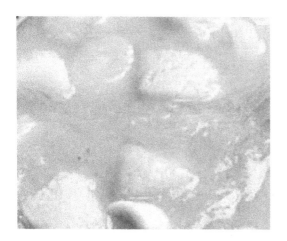

Ingredients

Ingredients Celeriac soup:

1 celeriac

Half root

1 onion (shallot)

1 clove of garlic

700 ml fat-free (chicken) broth

1 bunch of leaf parsley

Pam spray

Ingredients Chicken / beet salad:

2 chicken fillets

300 grams of beetroot

2 onions

dash of apple cider vinegar

2 tbsp lemon soup

Few twigs of dill

Salt and pepper

Preparation

Preparation of soup:

Slice the half carrot, chop the onion or shallot and finely chop the clove of garlic.

Cut the celeriac into large pieces.

Spray a little Pam spray in a saucepan and fry the onion, garlic and carrot.

After about 2 minutes, add the celeriac pieces and fry for a while. Then pour the stock over it and bring to the boil. Put a lid on the pan.

Reduce the heat a little and let it simmer for 20 minutes.

After 20 minutes you remove the pan from the heat and puree the whole until a lightly bound whole is created.

If desired, add a little pepper and salt and decorate the whole with leaf parsley.

Preparation of salad:

Cut the chicken into pieces and fry it in a pan. Then let it cool.

While cooling the chicken you can cut the red beets into small cubes. Snippe smoke the onion and finely chop the dill.

Put the cooled chicken and vegetables in a bowl and sprinkle with lemon juice and a dash of apple cider vinegar.

Season with pepper and salt.

SALAD WITH SHRIMP

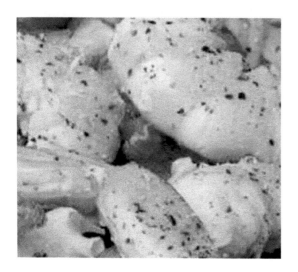

Ingredients

Mixed salad

8 prawns (or some shrimps)

1 clove of garlic

1 lime

1 red pepper

A little pepper and salt

Calve Salad Mix

Preparation

Preheat the oven to 180 degrees

Chop the garlic and put it on a sheet of baking paper.

Then cut the bell pepper into strips or cubes and place this with the chopped garlic.

Take the lime and cut it in half. Press the lime (juice) over the bell pepper and chopped garlic with your hands.

Finally, add the prawns and slide it all into the oven. Cook the whole in about 10 minutes.

In the meantime, take a bowl and add the mixed salad.

Make the salad tasty with the dressing (mix 1/4 bag of Calvé Salad Mix with a little water)

When the prawns are ready, you can mix this into the lettuce.

Season with a little pepper and salt.

Fish package with fennel

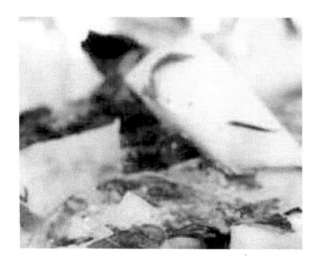

Ingredients

1 lemon

PEM spray

Fresh pepper and salt

2 fennel tubers

2 shallots

4 pieces of redfish fillet (approx. 110-130 grams each)

40 ml of dry white wine

Lettuce with snow peas

Aluminium foil

Preparation

Preheat the oven to 175 degrees.

Clean the lemon well and grate the zest. Spray Pem spray in a bowl and add the grated lemon zest and salt and pepper to taste. This is the lemon butter that we do over the fish.

Clean the fennel tubers and cut or scrape them into nice thin slices.

Also cut the shallots into small pieces.

Spread 4 pieces of approximately 50 cm of aluminum foil on your workbench.

Divide the sliced shallots and fennel slices in the middle of the pieces of foil. Put the fish on it and brush it in with the lemon butter.

Turn the foil into a sort of container and then pour a little wine next to the pieces of fish.

Fold the foil up and lay it on the baking tray in the oven.

Bake the fish in the oven for approximately 15 minutes.

Finally place the packages on a plate and carefully unfold them

Thai stir-fry

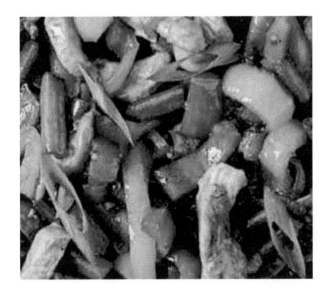

Ingredients

1 orange (or red) bell pepper

150 grams of snow peas

300 grams of shiitake

2 cloves of garlic

1 tbsp pepper rings

2 spring onions

200 grams of tuna

2 tbsp Thai fish sauce

1 lime

Iceberg lettuce

3 tbsp finely chopped coriander

Preparation

Start by boiling the snow peas in water with a little salt. Boil the snow peas for about 3 to 4 minutes until al dente. Then drain and rinse with cold water. Let it drain.

Meanwhile, chop the garlic, cut the spring onion into oblique rings, tear the shiitake into small pieces and cut the bell pepper into strips.

Heat a little PEM spray in the wok and fry the shiitake with the garlic for 2 to 3 minutes. Turn over the whole now and then.

Remove them from the pan and place them on a plate.

Heat the wok again and stir-fry the bell pepper, red pepper and spring onion. Let this bake for about 3 minutes.

Remove the pan from the heat and add the snow peas, the tuna, the fish sauce, the lime juice and the grater of the lime to the vegetables.

Season with a little pepper and salt to taste.

Divide iceberg lettuce over the plates and put the mixture on top.

Sprinkle with a little coriander.

Carpaccio with arugula

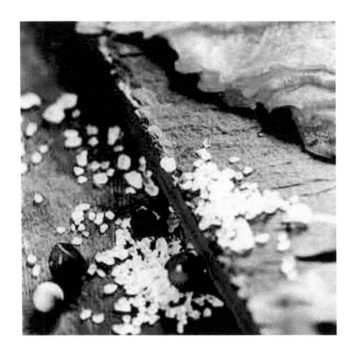

Ingredients

100 grams of beef carpaccio

Arugula

Sun dried tomatoes

Capers

Red onion

Balsamic vinegar

Pepper and salt

Fat-free broth

Preparation

Take a nice big plate and divide the thin slices of carpaccio over it.

Cut the red onion into smaller pieces and sprinkle over it.

Do this also with the sun-dried tomatoes and capers. If the sun-dried tomatoes are too large, you can first halve them.

To taste pepper, salt and the Balsamic vinegar

Oriental curry

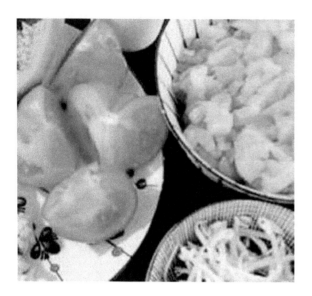

Ingredients

150 grams of chicken fillet

100 grams of low-fat yogurt

1 tsp curry

1 tsp coriander seed

1 tsp ginger

1 tsp honey

1 green pepper

1 tomato

1 red onion

about 20 grams of bean sprouts

Half a clove of garlic

salt

Pemspray

Preparation

Halve the bell pepper and onion. You will use the remaining halves later.

Cut the chicken fillet into cubes.

Take a pan and add the curry and coriander seeds. Put it on a high heat and bake the seeds brown (dry baking). This will give them more taste.

Pack a blender and add the tomato, half pepper, half onion, curry, coriander seeds, salt, ginger, honey and yogurt.

Blend everything until it is a nice sauce.

Put this sauce in a frying pan and cook the sliced chicken until tender.

Cut the other two halves of the bell pepper and onion into small pieces and fry them in another pan. Use a small amount of Pem Spray for this.

Finally, cook the bean sprouts. Not too long, because then it will become less crispy.

If the sauce is still a bit thin, you can tie it with a little cornflour.

Put the baked vegetables on a plate and spoon the chicken with sauce over it.

Cauliflower stew with Beef tartar

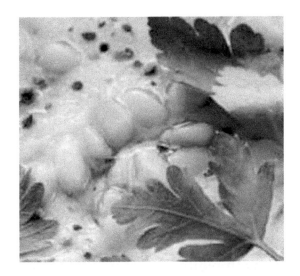

Ingredients

2 cauliflowers

200 grams of spinach

80 grams of sundried tomatoes

60 grams of blue cheese (light)

3 tablespoons pine nuts

A dash of milk

Pinch of nutmeg

Pepper and salt

PAM spray

4 beef tartars

Preparation method

Cut the cauliflower into florets. Then wash the roses well.

In the meantime, put a pan with plenty of water on the fire and bring to the boil. Put the florets in here and let it boil for about 10 minutes.

Then drain the cauliflower. Put the cooked cauliflower in a pan and add a dash of milk. Stamp the whole into a stew. If you want a smooth structure, you can puree it completely.

Season the cauliflower stew with a pinch of nutmeg and some salt and pepper.

Meanwhile, spray a baking pan with some PAM spray. Bake the beef tartlets in it.

Chop the spinach into large pieces and cut the sun-dried tomatoes into pieces. You can add this to the cauliflower stew.

Garnish the cauliflower stew with pine nuts and crumble some blue cheese over it.

Serve the stew with the beef tartare.

Lightning Source UK Ltd.
Milton Keynes UK
UKHW020647060421
381519UK00012B/878